SEX TIPS from a Dominatrix

PATRICIA PAYNE

Illustrations by MAURICE VELLEKOOP

ReganBooks

An Imprint of HarperCollins*Publishers*

SEX TIPS FROM A DOMINATRIX. Copyright © 1999 by Marthink. All rights reserved. Printed in the United States of America. No part of this book may be used or reproduced in any manner whatsoever without written permission except in the case of brief quotations embodied in critical articles and reviews. For information address HarperCollins Publishers, Inc., 10 East 53rd Street, New York, NY 10022.

HarperCollins books may be purchased for educational, business, or sales promotional use. For information please write: Special Markets Department, HarperCollins Publishers, Inc., 10 East 53rd Street, New York, NY 10022.

FIRST EDITION
Designed by Joseph Rutt

Illustrations for chapter openers by Maurice Vellekoop.
All other illustrations by Beth Trott.

ISBN 0-06-039287-8

99 00 01 02 01 ❖/RRD 10 9 8 7 6 5 4 3 2 1

To Charles Sego and Mary Beth Hebert

CONTENTS

Contents

Contents

Contents

ACKNOWLEDGMENTS

I would like to acknowledge Randy, Michael, and Lori (whips); Joyce (corsets); Cynthia (fashion); NoWannabes (electrical play); Chuck; Heather; Warren; my editor, Jeremie Ruby-Strauss, and all the women he will ever date; Doyle and the NY Yankees copier; Michelle; Lynn; Jan Marie; Gwenda; Janis; Hannah; and my mentor and domme de plume, Mistress Martha.

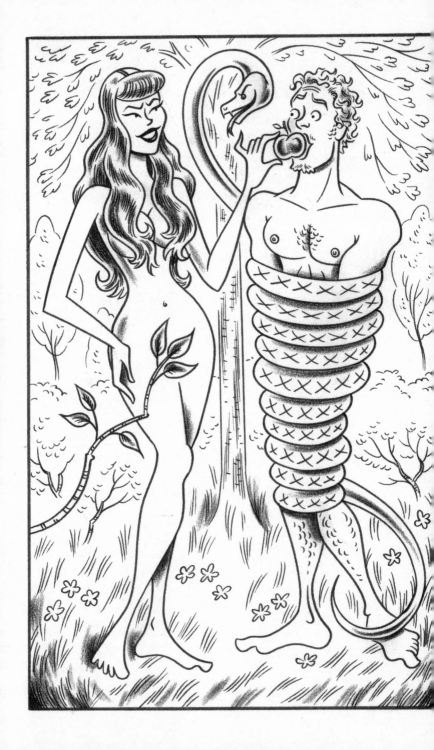

INTRODUCTION

"Samuel Adams, a taste you can stay tied up with all night," reads the tag line from a recent radio ad campaign from a very straitlaced Boston brewery. An episode of the prime-time phenomenon *Friends* has girl-next-door Lisa Kudrow breaking up a catfight between Jennifer Aniston and Courteney Cox. As she holds both of the kneeling combatants by the hair, she says, "I guess if we were in prison, you'd both be my bitches." Print media ads are glutted with glossy pictures of models in skin-tight latex, and every night, somewhere in syndication, Xena, fetish goddess, adjusts her bursting breastplates and cracks wise with her demurely submissive traveling companion about how much men dig the leather outfit.

Clearly, the times we live in are rife with allusion and innuendo to once deviant sexual practices, which even a few years ago would have been considered risqué at best and taboo at worst. Now, everyone giggles at the sitcom references to bondage and spanking, but underneath the laughter, do straight people secretly wonder if they are missing out on something? Why do references to the dark world of BDSM, (bondage/discipline, dominance/submission, sadism/masochism)[1] titillate us and coerce us into buying bottles of expensive vodka and tins of painfully peppery mints? What is it about bondage that would captivate a former president's daughter

---

1. There is some debate on the appropriate nomenclature for people who use the concept of power exchange for sexual gratification. For simplicity's sake, I will often use the terms *dominance and submission, bondage and discipline,* and *sadomasochism* (or their abbreviations, *D/s, B/D, S & M,* and the catch-all *BDSM* interchangeably and at my whim. This will also be true for words that describe people who participate in these activities: dominant, dominatrix, dom, domme, submissive, sub, top, bottom, owner, slave, master, and so on.

and *The General's Daughter*? Why would a mainstream *country* singer like Shania Twain show up to perform at the Grammy Awards in a custom corseted costume of towering heels and elbow-length gloves that was only missing a flogger and a pair of handcuffs?

Frankly, I don't care why. I am just delighted they do, for I am a practicing dominatrix: a woman who *has* masks, floggers, and handcuffs. I use my personal power over my sexual partner for our mutual erotic enjoyment. I am not concerned with the psychological ramifications of why this is enticing—just knowing that it *is* enticing is enough for me. I don't have to mess my manicure twisting wrenches on the engine of my Bentley to be able to drive it, nor do I have to milk a cow in order to serve ice cream. I am not a doctor (although I play one with TVs). I don't presume to understand the human mind nor the biological machinations of human sexual response. I *do* presume to notice, however, that when I cross my thigh-high-booted legs, every male head follows the movement in unison, like center-court spectators at Wimbledon. I do recognize the playful spark in a man's eyes when I tell him I think I will kidnap him for the weekend and have my way with him. I *see* him stand at attention when I trace a line down his chest with my crop.

As a dominatrix, I am more concerned with the how, what, and where of this errant eroticism. Humans have a luxury that other animals presumably don't have: the fantastic ability to create a storyline to their sexuality; to write their own amatory menu. If there is a *why* to be asked it is, indeed, "Why choose plain vanilla, when you can have the decadence of 'Death by Chocolate'?" *And* it's non-fattening.

Traditions and accoutrements embraced by the sado-masochistic community are the perfect embellishments for those wishing to add variety and flair to this most private part of their lives. In practicing dominance and submission, one is able to find rich traditions, intricate formalities, and a sense of order, even while being inventive. And, of course, seemingly endless paraphernalia—which is a good excuse for shopping, if nothing else. As I have often said, "a little dominance and submission in one's sex life is like a dash of cinnamon in potpourri."

To guide you through this brave new underworld, I will share with you some of my favorite tips I use for training and pleasuring my own submissives—a smorgasbord of little dishes from which you can pick and choose according to your own appetites. I will give you hints on how to introduce D/s—either as an hors d'oeuvre, an entrée, or a dessert—to your own sexual plate. In the pages that follow, I shall give you step-by-step instructions on how to choose a role, set the mood, decorate your room, pick a proper outfit, buy the best bonds, tie the exact knot, and wield the perfect quirt. Think of this as an erotic cookbook with the spiciest of recipes.

While part of its excitement is based on BDSM looking or even being dangerous, I will alert you to safety precautions to avoid trouble, accidents, and embarrassment. Certainly there exist extremists among practitioners, as there are in all walks of life, but the scene is not so much about pain and suffering as you may have been led to believe. The essence of S & M is not about historical oppression or pathological subjugation. It is about the consensual exchange of power that exists between sexual partners. It is about taking someone to the brink. About taking your lover to a blissed-out subspace enabled by the releasing of his control to you. Yes, D/s is about a love of bonds—but it is also about a bond of love. This cookbook is filled with recipes for pleasure rather than pain; for sweet things rather than bitter ones. It is about fun and D/lightfulness—a trip to D/sneyland.

So much of BDSM is beyond the hot clothing and cool equipment. As you perfect the techniques I describe, you will pick up more than just arcane erotic knowledge. You will notice a change in your overall bearing as you become more confident with your D/s persona. People, and especially men, will notice your new confidence in ways that are hard to quantify, but are nonetheless apparent. You will talk confidently and walk tall, with or without your stilettos. The tips in the following pages will give you the power to instill this mystery and the methods to install it as part of your own sexual psyche. Within these pages, you will learn to read, between the black and white lines, the deeper meaning of the black and blue.

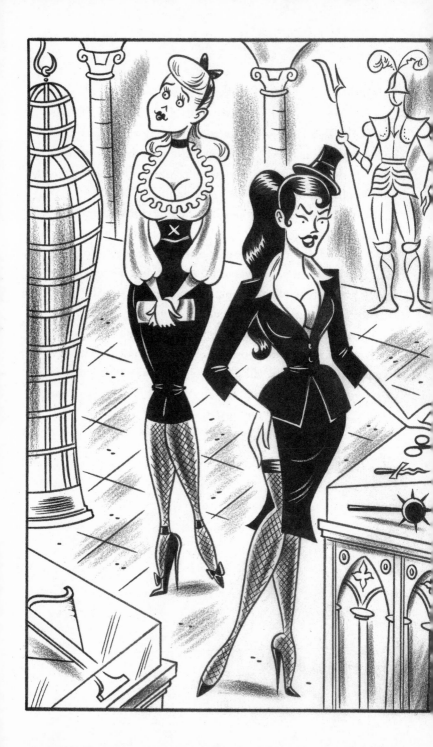

- 1 -

EMPOWERING OR ENSLAVING YOUR INNER CHILD

discovering your
dominance quotient

For some must follow and some command.
— LONGFELLOW

It has been said that there are two kinds of people in this world, people who think there are two kinds of people and people who don't. I maintain the world is made up of givers and takers, dominants and submissives, tops and bottoms—each pair in a symbiotic relationship like that between seamed stockings and stilettos.

The BDSM community is a place where desires you've only confessed to your best friend in her dorm room at Deerfield are perfectly acceptable. But whether you yearn to be a toy in a sensualist's FAO Schwartz or have a maid who can bring new meaning to "Her Majesty's Service," it is basic D/s protocol to be able to properly identify yourself as dominant or submissive.

This identification is critical because there is only one constant in a D/s relationship: one partner must have the dominant role, and one the submissive. If this basic guideline isn't followed, you will have two strong forces battling for control, or two submissive personalities clamoring to outdo each other in the rigors of service (a deplorable situation, although one that always leaves the bathroom immaculate).

d/scisions, d/scisions

Just as you must decide on chintz or silk for your curtains, so too must you decide whether to emphasize your dominant or submissive tendencies before you can become a player.

For some, this is an easy choice. My friend Dale once told me she realized she had submissive tendencies when she saw a spanking scene in a movie and it occurred to her she wanted to know what it felt like. I confessed I had had a similarly enlightening experience at the yacht club, but my reaction was "Wow, I have to learn how to tie that knot!"

For others, it may take some experimentation or soul searching to decide which side of the paddle they prefer. If a woman consistently chooses bikini waxing over a manicure, she has undeniable submissive tendencies. If she prefers using her Epilady, she is a full-fledged masochist. Or if a man always finds himself insisting that people refer to him as "Mr. Brown" or "Dr. Brown," that is an indication of his dominant nature, or at least a measure of the amount of stuffing in his shirt.

Having people identify items that best express their secret sexual longings can also be very telling, although some situations are trickier than others. I once knew a lovely couple from Newport who ran into difficulties when he donned a diaper and she a Catholic schoolgirl's skirt. It took a great deal of time, as well as a weekend submersion session of Lina Wertmuller films, before they were able to reach a symbiosis with the roles they had chosen.

domination 101

You have dominant tendencies if you are, or aspire to be, the prime orchestrator in the bedroom. However, good dominants should possess other important qualities.

Excellence in communication is one of the keys to being in control, and being in control is the key to being a good dominant. A good dominant states her preferences in a manner that is consistent, straightforward, and respectful. Similarly, she issues instructions in a clear, easy-to-understand manner.

A good working knowledge and willingness to learn the safe execution of BDSM activities is also an important characteristic of a dominant. She must be able to control her environment, her partner, and—most important—herself.

Dominants are no better than submissives, just different. Altruistic and compassionate to others, they understand that the world does not revolve around them. Except when it does.

trust you, truss me

You gotta serve somebody.
—BOB DYLAN

If you enjoy putting yourself out to do things for others, or if the thought of being instructed sexually makes you hot, you register on the submissive spectrum. This may be evidenced by heartfelt pleasure in serving your partner like a highly trained geisha or by sexual arousal when playing with sensory experiences like being tied up or spanked.

An educated submissive uses his head and not other libido-driven body parts when selecting a dominant, either for a BDSM scene or a relationship. This is critical because the sub must be able to trust his partner to safely lead him through the most formidable of BDSM activities.

Closely related to the ability to trust is a willingness to

obey. Debates about who is going to do what to whom and when is antithetical to the dynamic of a BDSM relationship. In addition, through obedience during play, a submissive takes an active role in ensuring his or her own safety.

Submissives must also have good communication skills (especially those "unspoken" ones). The more easily they can express their desires, fears, and limits to a dominant, the more likely they are to have a satisfying experience.

Submissive and needy are not synonymous. Most dominants do not wish to be your knight in shining armor 24/7.

would a domme by any other name swat as sweet?

The BDSM community has many different words for *dominant* and *submissive*. Here are some common terms and distinctions.

DOMINANT TYPES

DOMINANT (DOM/DOMME): The person in charge of a BDSM relationship. Dom is used when referring to a male dominant and domme to the female counterpart.

DOMINATRIX: A female, sometimes professional, dominant.

MASTER/MISTRESS: Respective male and female terms for an experienced dominant. These terms are also used when referring to a dominant significant other in a BDSM relationship. For example, "I bought Master a new flogger last week," or "Tell your mistress I found you to be very well behaved."

SADIST: A person who enjoys giving pain.

TOP: A person who sexually dominates a submissive, but does not control other aspects of their relationship.

SUBMISSIVE TYPES

BOTTOM: A person who is submissive during a BDSM scene, but not within the other aspects of a relationship.

SUBMISSIVE (SUB): A person who surrenders physical and mental control within an intimate BDSM relationship, but is generally independent and in control of his or her life otherwise (unless she is a woman trying to get the remote control from her lover).

SLAVE: A person who feels an intense level of submission toward his or her dominant partner, often within the context of a live-in relationship. Sometimes used synonymously for *submissive*.

MASOCHIST: A person who enjoys receiving pain.

SAM (SMART-ASS MASOCHIST): A masochist or bottom who deliberately provokes a dominant; a brat.

OTHER TYPES

LEATHERMAN/WOMAN: The segment of the gay and lesbian community that practices BDSM.

SWITCH: Switches enjoy both dominant and submissive roles. They are excellent people to know if your dungeon party has too many guests of one predilection or another.

"yes, sir, domme"

What's in a name? That which we call a rose
By any other name would smell as sweet.
—SHAKESPEARE

People often ask me to clear up their confusion about nomenclature in the sadomasochistic community. Are all masters doms? Is a submissive the same as a slave? Why did the masochist refuse to tie me up?

Like the federal tax codes, there are no hard and fast rules. And like food labeling, there isn't any regulating mechanism in place to keep D/s players from pretty much calling themselves anything they like.

The first thing to remember is, as with other appellations, there are those words that are titular and those that are descriptive. Titular words such as *Lord* or *Master* are the most confusing for beginners, for just like vintners from Bordeaux, people are forever attaching their names to those who have achieved success or renown.

Players often have their own highly thought out and personal reasons for why they choose to call themselves *Mistress* over *Madam*, but beginners need only remember one thing: nine out of ten times, people who use a title are dominant. Keeping this in mind will help you find the partner of your dreams, whether it be online or at a club or social event. While some dominants prefer that their bottoms address them by their particular title, unless you are told otherwise, think of *Dom, Mistress,* and *Sir* as being equivalent.

If you enter into a relationship or even a one-spank stand

with a dominant, a good rule of thumb is that as in everything else, dominants are called as they wish to be, and call submissives as they wish to.

On the other hand, descriptive appellations can be a major help in understanding what an individual's preferences are. Masters, doms, mistresses, and tops all have one thing in common. They will expect their partners to willingly yield to them. Similarly, subs, slaves, and bottoms are all people who surrender control.

Members of the gay community who also enjoy the nuances of sadomasochism have their own nomenclature. The terms *leatherman* and *leatherwoman* are generic identifiers, whereas some female dominants like to be called *Daddy*, just as some male submissives respond well to *Boy*.

While a rose by any other name may smell as sweet, a mistress who is asked to kneel may forever hold a grudge, so it is important part of D/s etiquette to keep these basic guidelines in mind.

Here is a simple quiz to help you determine if you are dominant or submissive. This should save you hours of introspection and permit you to get on to the most important part of D/s, the shopping . . . I mean, the sex. Be comfortable with your results, and remember, unlike being locked into that dreadful time share in Hilton Head, you can always change your mind.

d/tails:
are you dominant or submissive?

1. You're at a restaurant with six other people and there is some question as to who will order first. You . . .
   a) patiently wait until it's your turn.
   b) order first, just for you.
   c) order for the whole table.
   d) peel the gag off your girlfriend and have her say, "The usual for my master."

2. While getting a rectal exam, you . . .
   a) get really disgusted.
   b) wonder if you will ever be able to get aroused again.
   c) moan, as usual.
   d) back into the finger.

3. You are walking by a hardware store. Something in the window catches your eye . . .
   a) Some PVC piping.
   b) The chain on the snow tire.
   c) The clothespins on the laundry rack.
   d) The hooks holding the sign up.

4. In your Range Rover, you . . .
   a) never wear a seat belt.
   b) always wear a seat belt.

c) pull the seat belt extra tight.
d) wrap the seat belt around your ankles and
wrists, too.

5. Going through your closet, looking for something to
wear to a wedding, your color choices are . . .
a) faded black.
b) black.
c) brand new black.
d) black leather.

6. You are on a job interview. Your potential boss says
he wants someone to run his life. You . . .
a) hand him the personals from this week's
alternative paper.
b) give him your mother's phone number.
c) have him put his feet flat on the floor with his
hands spread on the table.
d) peel down to your leather underwear and start
scrubbing the floor.

7. If you had to pick a celebrity dom role model you are
most like, it would be . . .
a) Charlton Heston.
b) Charles Bronson.
c) Prince Charles.
d) Charles Nelson Reilly.

8. While on a dinner date, your partner says "Feed me."
   You . . .
   a) slip her a forkful of spaghetti.
   b) order "Death by Chocolate" and two spoons.
   c) slip her a forkful of champagne.
   d) fall to your knees between her legs and then say,
      "Oh, I thought you said 'Eat me.'"

9. Your favorite scotch is . . .
   a) Chivas.
   b) Dewars.
   c) Pinch.
   d) Cutty.

10. If you had to pick a celebrity domme role model you
    are most like, it would be . . .
    a) June Cleaver.
    b) Cher.
    c) Madonna.
    d) Cruella De Ville.

11. You are deciding on a new hobby and are leaning
    toward . . .
    a) macramé.
    b) leathercraft.
    c) witchcraft.
    d) body piercing.

12. The metal detector at the airport goes off from . . .
    a) your pocket flashlight.
    b) your nipple clamp.
    c) your handcuffs.
    d) your chastity belt.

13. While you're asleep, your apartment is broken into.
    You . . .
    a) insist on being tied up.
    b) help pick matching scarves for your gag.
    c) complain that you can reach the knot.
    d) boast that your handcuffs are better.

14. When you scan the personal ads in your local paper,
    the words that catch your eye are . . .
    a) long walks.
    b) long walks on the beach.
    c) long walks on the beach in heels.
    d) long walks on the beach in shackles.

15. You are at the race track and you . . .
    a) wonder how many jockeys it would take to serve
       you.
    b) can't help but notice if you stacked two jockeys,
       their mouths would be in the nicest places.
    c) wonder if the harnesses come in a size 2.
    d) are impressed the gag bits match your Guccis.

16. Your date asks you to do "The Whip." You . . .
    a) are disappointed that she is referring to the name of the dance.
    b) request more bare backs.
    c) wonder where the damn whip is?
    d) put in a request to dance "The Crop" next.

17. You have a $50 gift certificate to a pet store. You . . .
    a) wonder if $50 would cover the stud fee for a really large Great Dane.
    b) buy a gerbil.
    c) make a deposit on a steel cage large enough for your lover.
    d) buy a dog collar although you own a blue-tip Siamese.

18. You are going backpacking and can pack only one pair of shoes. You take . . .
    a) hiking boots.
    b) motorcycle boots.
    c) mules.
    d) stiletto heels.

19. You are named the chairperson of a major fund-raising ball. The theme you choose is . . .
    a) Arabian Nights.
    b) Easy Rider.
    c) Betty Page: The Irwin Klaw Years.
    d) The Spanish Inquisition.

20. Your most generous term of affection is:
    a) Babe.
    b) Kissy-toes.
    c) Master.
    d) Panty-slut.

KEY:

If you scanned over up to five questions, then went on to something else, you have strong dom tendencies.

If you read more than five items, but did not keep track of your score, you have moderate dom tendencies.

If you read the whole quiz, answered some questions, and then skipped ahead to read this, you have moderate sub tendencies.

If you read and answered all questions, and did not look at this key until you had permission to do so, you have strong sub tendencies.

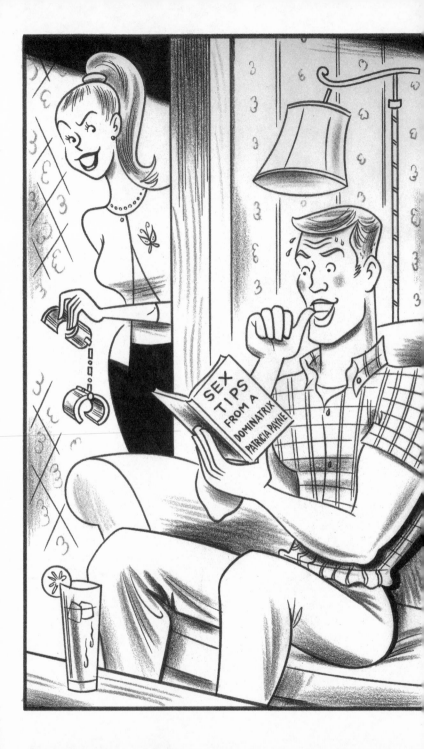

- 2 -
AN INVITATION
TO INEQUITY

introducing bdsm
to your partner

*Being your slave, what should I do but tend upon the
hours and times of your desire?*
—SHAKESPEARE

Your domme box is packed with clothespins and ribbon;
you've purchased a Vivienne Westwood bustier and a pair of
patent Manolos; you have more crops than Iowa has corn . . .
how to spring this on your partner?

Introducing BDSM as part of your passion palate need
not be as daunting a proposition as it appears. Unless your
partner is known for loving full-blown, quirky surprises,
don't start out by converting your den into a dungeon.
Instead, start down this path by taking small steps that let
him know where your interests lie. Fortunately for you, day-
to-day life presents a multitude of opportunities to subtly
expose your partner to your wildest fantasies.

The idea of assuming or relinquishing control in a sexual
context appeals to many people and can range from the simple
"I'd like you to wear your sexy underwear tonight" to "How
'bout if you make me your sex slave this weekend?" Remember
that even the most vanilla of traditional sex acts have an element of power exchange, so it's not like you are treading on
uncharted territory. The single most important first step is to
steel yourself against the possibility of getting rebuffed.

If you are already in a relationship, clear your channels of
communication like you would your calendar for those days
at the Ranch and have an earnest conversation with your

partner. You may discover there is a sexual piranha lurking under that Brooks Brother's clothing.

Inventory how you and your partner interact and what aspects of these interactions you find the most satisfying. If your partner often takes the initiative doing things for you, chances are good that he or she will like being *told* what to do for you. Remember to always be gracious and polite when issuing your orders; you are a dominant, not Leona Helmsley. Conversely, if you are feeling submissive, consider giving your partner a card offering your services as personal servant for an evening.

seeing is believing

No matter what you are doing, your choice of clothing can help set a tone and send a strong message as to your dominant or submissive leanings. Women don't have to wear leather and carry a bullwhip to project the air of a dominatrix. A simple, dark, tailored suit paired with a pair of four-inch pumps will work almost as well. Accessories, such as gloves, convey a mild kinkiness. Women's hairstyles, such as being slicked back in early Annie Lennox style or pulled back into a severe bun, can convey a D/s message while simultaneously being perfectly respectable and appropriate. (This kind of hairstyle also functions as a temporary face lift.) Men who are interested in submitting can covertly signal their interests by wearing a pair of linen pants with no underwear. (What's more revealing, especially if he is just the slightest bit aroused?)

Coffee-table books not only add an air of elegance to your love nest, but can be great conversation starters, too.

Buy a copy of *Fetish Girls*, by Eric Kroll, and casually leave it out in the living room. Then find an excuse to leave the room long enough that your guest is forced to look around to entertain himself. If you are very lucky, you will return to find him with book in hand, and you have the perfect opening. If not, wait a while to see if he mentions it, or you can find some way to work it into the conversation. On the off chance your guest is put off by such racy material, say it was a gift and you've left it out so as not to offend the giver.

"and the bondy award goes to . . ."

There's no casual date more commonplace than renting a film. And it just so happens there are lots of very good mainstream films with BDSM scenes or themes, so you can dispense with any fears you might have about appearing pervy to your partner. As an added bonus, these movies will spare you a trip to the local adult video store, where you spend all your time worrying about getting something yucky on your trench coat while you peruse the aisles.

Use the moments that present themselves during the movie to bring up a desire of yours. Look into your partner's eyes, plant a soul-shattering kiss, and say something like, "I couldn't help but think how sweet you would look tied and gagged like Madeleine Stowe." This is also a great time to suggestively play with the hairline on his neck or trace a line up his calf with the toe of your high-heeled pump.

More graphic films, such as *9 1/2 Weeks*, can open the door a little wider. If your partner is clearly interested in Kim

Basinger's enslavement, take a bathroom break and strip down to something sexy. You can leave your hat on.

d/tails:
twenty bdsm movies
you can rent almost
anywhere

9 1/2 Weeks (1986), starring Mickey Rourke, Kim Basinger; directed by Adrian Lyne.

    Kim Basinger increasingly becomes Mickey Rourke's sex slave over a period of . . . you know.

Behind the Green Door (1972), starring Marilyn Chambers, George McDonald; directed by Art and Jim Mitchell.

    This is one of the few hard-core porn movies ever to become recognized as a major film, a tribute to its professional photography and Marilyn Chambers's "can-do" attitude.

Belle De Jour (1967) starring Catherine Deneuve, Jean Sorel, Michel Piccoli; directed by Luis Buñuel.

    Catherine Deneuve plays a bored housewife who has sadomasochistic fantasies and moonlights at a brothel. Plus, it's French!

The Black Glove (1996), starring Maria Beatty, Mistress Morgan; directed by Jay Bliznick.

    A silent, black-and-white short that depicts a David Lynch–like BDSM scene between a domme and her female submissive.

Body of Evidence (1993), starring Madonna, Willem Dafoe, Joe Mantegna, Anne Archer; directed by Uli Edel.

A film noir with Madonna and a hot (no pun intended) waxing scene. How could you not love a movie with the line, "You will see she is not only the defendant, she is the murder weapon itself"?

Bound (1996), starring Jennifer Tilly, Gina Gershon; directed by Andy and Larry Wachowski.

Girls swindle a counterfeiter, explore girl-girl sex, and get tied up a lot, especially the streetwise butch lesbian played by Gershon.

Boxing Helena (1993), starring Julian Sands, Sherilyn Fenn; directed by Jennifer Chambers Lynch.

Another interesting movie about the importance of power in a relationship. Fenn also adds a unique flair to voyeurism.

Bull Durham (1988), starring Kevin Costner, Susan Sarandon, Tim Robbins; directed by Ron Shelton.

Your guy will love this movie because it's about baseball and because most men think Susan Sarandon is hot. You'll love this because Tim Robbins in stockings and a garter is worth a $2.50 movie rental and because Sarandon's character is domme subtle at its finest.

The Collector (1965), starring Terence Stamp, Samantha Eggar; directed by William Wyler.

A kidnapping thriller that examines the bond that develops between a kidnapper and his hostage.

Exit to Eden (1994), starring Rosie O'Donnell, Dan Aykroyd, Dana Delany; directed by Garry Marshall.

It's not very erotic and it's not very funny. But if you're into BDSM, it could be Eden to you.

The Fountainhead (1949), starring Gary Cooper, Patricia Neal; directed by King Vidor.

Forget about that dreary plot about self-actualization and architecture. The Roark/Francon relationship is a classic example of power exchange. Everyone smokes and wears hats.

Last Tango in Paris (1973), starring Marlon Brando, Maria Schneider; directed by Bernardo Bertolucci.

This movie has hot sex, a relatively thin Marlon Brando, and two Academy Award nominations, allowing you to be simultaneously kinky and erudite.

Maîtresse (1976), starring Gérard Depardieu, Bulle Ogier; directed by Barbet Schroeder.

A young, buff Depardieu breaks into a dominatrix's apartment; after she catches him, he becomes her slave.

McLintock! (1963), starring John Wayne, Maureen O'Hara; directed by Andrew V. McLaglen.

John Wayne is actually funny in this movie. The famous spanking scene was a cinematic first.

The Nightcomers (1972), starring Marlon Brando, Stephanie Beacham; directed by Michael Winner.

Based on the Henry James short story "The Turn of the Screw"; Marlon Brando plays a gardener involved in a sadomasochistic relationship with the nurse of two rich orphans.

The Night Porter (1973), starring Dirk Bogarde, Charlotte Rampling; directed by Liliana Cavani.

A sadomasochistic bond is rekindled between a hotel's night porter, a former concentration camp officer, and a guest, his victim/lover from the past.

Seven Beauties (1976), starring Giancarlo Giannini, Shirley Stoler; directed by Lina Wertmuller.
Wertmuller received an Academy Award nomination for Best Director for this film about the sadomasochistic relationship that develops between a concentration camp matron and an inmate who has been separated from his seven ghastly sisters.

Swept Away (1975), starring Giancarlo Giannini, Mariangela Melato; directed by Lina Wertmuller.
Bitch on boat. Worker on boat. Boat wreck. Island. Tables are turned. She digs him, asks him to sodomize her (he doesn't know the meaning of the word). Rescue. Back to her world. Best viewed as a double feature with *Seven Beauties*.

Unforgiven (1992), starring Clint Eastwood, Gene Hackman, Morgan Freeman, Richard Harris; directed by Clint Eastwood.
Yes, Clint Eastwood deserved all the Academy Awards for his depiction of a cowboy antihero. But forget that. What about that flogging scene?

Whispering Smith (1948), starring Alan Ladd, Brenda Marshall; directed by Leslie Fenton and Mel Epstein.
A pretty nondescript cowboy-detective movie that also has one hell of a flogging scene.

dinner and immovie

You can also combine food with your film for that time-tested date routine of dinner and a movie, especially in these days of video dates where you can dine and view in the privacy of your own home. Think about an exquisite meal of erotically suggestive food where you coquettishly offer to feed your pet. This gets him used to having things put in his mouth, while at the same time, he relinquishes more power to you. When you finish your Tom Jonesian bacchanalia, you can turn down the lights and turn on the home theater.

If you enjoy clubbing, take your partner to a Goth club. The Goth scene has a strong BDSM undercurrent to it. Fetish clothing enjoys a high popularity, and BDSM toys like floggers, paddles, and handcuffs are also highly visible, though most commonly used as accessories. The music is loud and frequently suggestive, so it's a great time to grab your partner and wiggle provocatively on the dance floor.

You can also add a sense of adventure and gambling to your tennis matches and video games by making a little D/s wager on the side: "Eight ball in the corner pocket, and you get tied to the bed tonight." Bondage poker makes for some interesting bets as well. A couple I know took their love of Trivial Pursuit to new levels with their version of "Bondage Jeopardy." I'll take "Potent Potables" for the handcuffs, Alex.

Be it subtle or overt, role play can also be used to add an element of power exchange to your interactions. The idea of being punished for doing something naughty is a hot trigger for many people and one that is easily introduced in the course of your normal interactions.

This is a perfect time to make charm school pay off. Observing the slightest breach in etiquette can provide you with an opportunity to instruct, improve, and properly punish the transgressor. A more elaborate variation on this is fantasy role play. There is an endless list of hero and villain roles and costumes for you to chose from, from pirate and captured damsel to Ken Starr and Monica Lewinsky. Sometimes, real-life situations lead to fantasy applications. More than one equestrian has been aroused by the boots, spurs, and smell of leather associated with riding horses.

If you have a dominant personality, don't be afraid to take advantage of the lowered resistance that often arises in the heat of passion. See how your partner responds to having his hands pinned over his head, or to a light tug on his hair or ears. Or render him speechless by placing your hand over his mouth.

One word of caution: because BDSM is rooted in mutual trust and submission, it inevitably makes people feel closer and more intimate. It is not something you casually introduce to the person you picked up at a bar an hour ago. Use these tricks to break the routine, not someone's heart.

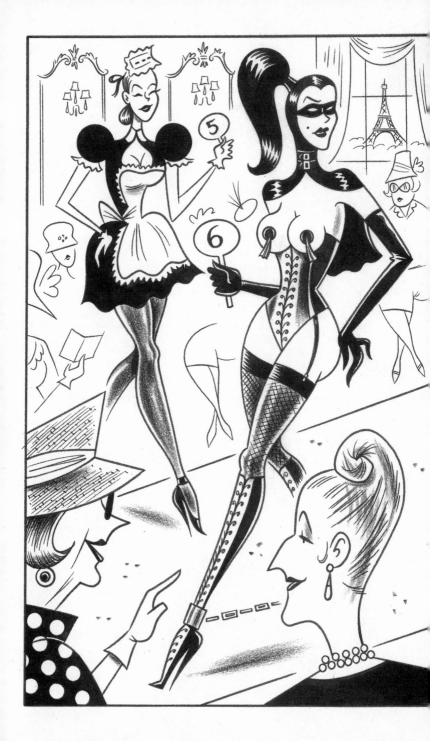

- 3 -

DRESSING WELL, THE BEST REVENGE

better on the rack
than off the rack

Dress to look your best, but first learn what is best for you. Step outside of yourself and regard your reflection as a stranger you are meeting for the first time.
—JANE DERBY

When I reflect on the importance of fashion in my life, I am apt to recall Ralph Waldo Emerson's observation, "The sense of being perfectly well-dressed gives a feeling of inner tranquillity which religion is powerless to bestow." If the world of D/s is where you wish to reside, or at least visit, then fashion must be your calling card. From the stern black leather pants of a dominant to the frilly lace of a submissive maid, choosing the correct clothing helps create a visual statement about your sexuality.

Clothing adds to your environment in the same way the right props complement a theatrical production, or the perfect wine can turn a commonplace dinner into something memorable. Imagine a scenario where a sadistic dominant is dressed in madras shorts, a Bub's BBQ T-shirt, black socks, and sneakers while the submissive is turned out in a Demask bustier and a pair of Manolo Blahnik shoes—suddenly it's clear how attire can backfire.

In most of our daily lives, circumstance dictates what we wear. We put on Lycra to go to the gym, a suit to go to the office, and shorts and a polo shirt for a Sunday afternoon picnic. But late at night, when the lights go down and the beeswax candles are lit, it is time for clothing that announces our mood, availability, or preference.

Fetish wear can be generally thought of as clothing to inspire the senses. I like to classify it as visual, tactile, and olfactory—or, to paraphrase Anthony Burgess, viddies, feelies, and smellies.

appearances can be demeaning

While revealing or slinky attire is not mandatory in order to participate in BDSM activities, having a general sense of what to wear can help make you feel more comfortable (in the same way wearing tie-dye at a Grateful Dead concert contributed to your feeling like one of the crowd). As you first start out, focus on looking your best and being comfortable. No one is expecting you to switch from Laura Ashley to Jean-Paul Gaultier overnight, so take your time as you assemble your fetish clothing collection. There is a wide range of materials, designs, and colors to chose from, and with due diligence, you are certain to find the appropriate articles for creating your ideal, individual fashion statement.

While this chapter focuses on fashion, it should be noted that nothing says vulnerability and submission like nudity. How an individual responds to being naked tells us a great deal about him. Modest or proud, apologetic or laissez-faire, when we are naked, our posture becomes our clothing and fashion statement.

living in a material world

There is no denying that some materials, especially those with a glossy surface or a soft, slippery texture, have an erotic appeal. Silk, satin, and velvet are appropriate for any D/s occasion, and fetish garments made from these fabrics require no more attention than you would give to day-to-day clothing cut from the same cloth. Other materials, such as leather and latex, may be new to your wardrobe, and you need to be aware these fabrics have qualities that merit special care and consideration.

leather

Except for vegetarians, black leather is *the* fashion staple of the BDSM community. Leather is suitable for many garments, from bras and jock straps to vests and chaps, as well as shoes and gloves. As dyeable as most fabric, leather is remarkably versatile and can accommodate any mood. Its many grades make it affordable for even those on a tight budget, but the soft, buttery feel of fine Italian leather is unparalleled. Properly treated leather will last for years, and with a little polish, takes on a luxurious sheen. Patent leather, my personal favorite, combines an incomparable shine with the heady smell of cowhide.

Leather is also the perfect material for many of the preferred implements for dominance and submission, like crops, whips, blindfolds, handcuffs . . . the list is almost endless, and matching leather clothing and accoutrements are as sound an investment as your favorite blue-chip stock.

caring for your hide

While leather is an attractive and resilient material, special care should be used to keep your hide in top shape.

An easy and simple step I always take after wearing leather clothing is to run a lint-free cloth over it, which keeps the dirt and dust out of the pores and creases of the garment. Remember to never condition your leather before cleaning, or you will simply seal in dirt and grime.

While a good dry cleaner is worth its weight in platinum, thorough cleaning of your leather clothing is something you can easily do at home—and it saves money (for more D/s shopping). Begin this process by applying saddle soap, following the manufacturer's instructions. After this cleaning process is complete, keep your leather from cracking and drying by applying Neet's Foot Oil to it.

Many leather garments come lined with either silk or nylon to keep the seams from chafing your skin. Silk linings can be cleaned by applying diluted Woolite with a damp sponge and then rinsing with another clean, damp sponge. Clean nylon linings by generously applying Woolite Spray Foam Upholstery Cleaner. Once the nylon is dry, the detergent is easily removed with a hand vacuum cleaner or a regular vacuum with a hose attachment.

Always be sure to store your leather in a clean, dry place. While plastic can be fun, plastic bags should be avoided as a storage option for your leather clothing. Plastic retains moisture, especially if you live in a humid area, and porous leather requires free-circulating air.

You may have noticed that well-loved and oft-worn

leather garments tend to stretch out at pressure points such as the knees, derriere, and elbows. Before donating your stretched-out frock to a slightly less fit friend, try shrinking it back to its original fit: Place the garment between two cotton towels and set an iron to medium heat. Iron over the towel for a few minutes and then try it on. Repeat as necessary until it fits the way you would like it to.

d/tails:
men, are you too old for
leather pants?

When I see people dressed in hideous clothes that look all wrong on them, I try to imagine the moment they were buying them and thought, "This is great. I like it. I'll take it."

—ANDY WARHOL

A special note to male dominants: Mistress Payne sympathizes with your seeming lack of fashion options. However, there is life beyond black jeans and matching black T-shirts. Riding attire, police or military uniforms (dress only), tuxes, even the Zorro look, can have a powerful effect on a submissive and add to your already powerful and domineering aura. The one fashion faux pas you must be sure to avoid is wearing leather pants when it is inappropriate for you to do so.

Note the sad case of Pat Boone, who raised so many eyebrows when he chose to not only put out a heavy metal album but also, in the spirit of the genre, do some publicity shots and appearances in black leather. While many of his longtime Christian followers were dismayed by his seeming allegiance with the devil, I believe there should have been a louder outcry against a man of his age wearing leather pants.

Use the following guide to help you determine when it is time to turn those trousers into seat covers. Employ your strongest personal critique to determine where on each of these scales you would fit to the degree you would be considered sexually desirable to a horny twenty-year-old waitress.

Elvis at twenty-five is the perfect leather horse. Fat, fortyish Elvis on downers should leave the building.

STUDLINESS	POINTS
1) Woody Allen, Pee-wee Herman	1
2) Bill Clinton, Bob Dole	2
3) Alan Alda, Robin Williams	5
4) Donald Trump, Hillary Clinton	10
5) Sly Stallone, Tom Cruise	20

RESPECTABILITY	
1) Banker, Lawyer	2
2) Wino, Bookie	4
3) Dentist, Architect	5
4) Clerk, Cabbie	10
5) Bartender, Trucker	15

AGE

1) Puberty–21	10
2) 22–29	15
3) 30–39	8
4) 40–54	4
5) 55+	2

HIPNESS

1) Rush Limbaugh, Goofy	1
2) Al Gore, Prince Charles	2
3) Michael Douglas, Eddie Murphy	6
4) Timothy Leary, Sting	10
5) Elvis Presley, Kurt Cobain	20

To obtain your score, multiply the points from each of the four categories.

TOTAL =

(Studliness) × (Respectability) × (Age) × (Hipness)

scoring:

1–500: Cowhide is out of the question.

501–1000: Become thinner or younger and leather will be OK.

1001–10,000: Wear them now, you won't be able to in ten years.

10,001+: Call me for a fitting.

sample scores:
Young Elvis: $10 \times 15 \times 15 \times 20 = 45,000$
James Dean: $20 \times 4 \times 15 \times 10 = 12,000$
Sixteen-year-old garage-band studmuffin:
$10 \times 10 \times 10 \times 2 = 2,000$
Bill Clinton: $2 \times 2 \times 4 \times 5 = 80$
Bill Gates: $1 \times 2 \times 8 \times 1 = 16$
Rush Limbaugh: $1 \times 2 \times 4 \times 1 = 8$

skin, too

Women should dress to give pleasure to men and pain to other women.

—HENRY WISE MILLER

Nothing says constriction like rubber and its relative PVC. If you can't bind your love with your favorite white cotton sash cord, you can make him almost as helpless and appealing by restricting him in a form-fitting rubber or PVC wardrobe.

Rubber has a unique ability to accentuate ambient temperature. To put it simply, if you are strutting your stuff on the dance floor or a crowded dungeon, you will quickly become hotter than you look, and under that form-fitting dress there will be a completely lubricated surface.

Rubber and latex are both products of the *Heva brasiliensis,* a type of rubber tree, and are the vegetarian's leather. Latex has a lighter gauge than rubber, so it is stretchier and easier to make into form-fitting apparel. While latex has a universal appeal, some people are allergic to it, so a considerate dominant will always ask her pet if he has ever had any adverse reactions to latex gloves or condoms before spending a bundle on her bundle. If latex is problematic, polyvinyl chloride (PVC), a synthetic rubber, is a great substitute (and so popular, it is almost mainstream). A PVC dress will be lighter than the same design in latex, but will have a similar sheen. It doubles as a perfect raincoat, and by making it skin tight in places, you can transform yourself into a perfect DominMatrix.

While there is nothing like latex to show off the fabulous figure you and your personal trainer work so hard to maintain, there are special considerations you should keep in mind as you dress for distress.

As you are certain to remember from advanced-placement chemistry, latex and petroleum are both hydrocarbons, so any oil-based compound that comes in contact with latex will cause it to disintegrate. To avoid this, don't use any petroleum-based products like lotion on your skin before wearing latex. Instead, apply a light dusting of unscented talcum powder to both your skin and all internal surfaces of the garment before putting it on.

While there is never an excuse for unkempt fingernails, a good manicure is de rigueur before donning any latex article. Sharp objects, like a broken nail, can easily puncture this delicate fabric. You should also remove any jewelry that can potentially snag your clothing.

To get the incredible sheen latex is known for, I suggest using Armor All or silicone spray for the ultimate in slick and shiny, although one should never apply these in rooms with tiled or marbled floors (unless you are willing to risk a shiner with your shine). I always use a lint-free cloth to spread and buff the latex and to prevent my garments from looking speckled. Beware that rubbing too hard with a cloth can damage the surface of the garment. Silicone can also be a little sticky, so any well-appointed slave to fashion should steer clear of rubbing against Grandmama's Irish linen tablecloth for fear of walking away with it and the Waterford in tow.

Latex stockings can perk up many an ensemble, but no matter how glamorous your gams, they have an annoying tendency to roll down. I do not recommend garters, as they can tear the fabric, but the adhesive that football players use on their hands during practice is water-soluble and, coincidentally, keeps your latex leggings firmly in place.

Removing your latex clothing while you are showering is a sensuous experience that is also good for your garments. Use a pure, unscented soap, and the sweat and body oils that are the archenemies of latex will wash away. Hang your clothing to dry or lay flat with nothing on top of it (turn it inside out to dry the other side). Once dry, lightly dust it with more unscented talcum powder, hang it on an untreated, preferably wooden hanger, and store it away from the light. Never store latex and leather clothing next to each other, as conditions that are good for leather destroy latex.

Even with the best of care, accidents do happen, and while your bichon frise certainly did not mean to nip and tear at the hem of your dress, his mark may appear to be indelible. An inner-tube repair kit is a simple, economical, and handy way to repair small tears in latex. If your garment is not black, cut a small piece from a passé latex dress or corset whose color matches the tear and use that for your patch. Rubber cement also works wonders on any seams that may become unglued.

all's well that ends well

*Fashion is only the attempt to realize Art in living forms
and social intercourse.*

—Oliver Wendell Holmes

To help you get started on planning your ensemble, let us begin
with Da Vinci's Vitruvian Man, which I have slightly improved
on. As fetishes are most commonly associated with the body's
extremities, working from the top down, select an appropriate
item of apparel for each asset to be emphasized. By simply
choosing the appropriate hat or headgear, gloves, and shoes, you
can build the rest of your ensemble around these items.

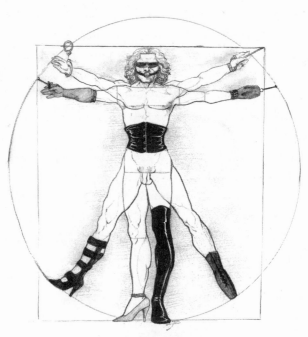

hats

*A hat is the difference between wearing clothes and
wearing a costume; it's the difference between being
dressed and dressed up; it's the difference between
looking adequate and looking your best.*
—MARTHA SALTER

Hats are an oft-overlooked apparel item, yet there are few
things that will distinguish you from the rest of the crowd
like a proper topper. Millinery stores are coming back into
vogue, and there are a wide variety of styles to suit any head
and occasion. Always make sure to look in a full-length mirror before making a purchase to ensure your hat is in pro-
portion to the rest of your body. A dominant may also want
to consider hoods, masks, or gags as acceptable substitutes
for a submissive's chapeau.

gloves

Well-appointed dominants should never leave the house
without a good pair of gloves, and short black leather gloves
should be a standard item for any dom. However, I like to
encourage dommes to have a variety of gloves in different
lengths, fabrics, and colors. Gloves are not only a perfect extremity accentuation, but, with a little creativity and a good knot, they
can be used to make an excellent impromptu gag or blindfold.

corsets

Corsets are one of the most popular fetish items, for they
have the combined appeal of both constriction and body

modification. Corset training follows the age-old tradition of modifying a person's mind, body, and spirit through waist constriction. Victorian women considered tight lacing virtuous, and that belief remains with us today, as many masters consider a loose corset a certain sign of a submissive in need of more training. The tight strictures of a corset make getting undressed a long and difficult task, perfect for putting your bottom on the brink of pleasure and leaving her (or him) there for a while. Corseting is also a wonderful way to keep your submissive looking great and is certainly preferable to Weight Watchers. Over time, a careful master can shape his submissive's figure into a picture-perfect hourglass, like a gardener carefully pruning a Bonsai tree.

Corsets make a perfect wardrobe staple, as the endless variety of colors and fabrics are enough to please the most fickle of fashion divas. They range from socially acceptable haute couture to devices that are best for intimate home-training situations. A cleverly made corset is suitable for formal evening wear, while at the same time it provides a submissive with a constant reminder of her dominant's grip (even if his hands are actually on his cell phone and martini).

Corseting enthusiasts have three basic body shapes to choose from: the classic hourglass (full hips and a cinched waist), the wasp waist (a long, narrow torso) and the most severe modification, the ice-cream cone (combining the full hips of the hourglass with the elongated torso of the wasp waist).

The proper fitting of a corset is very important. No one wants a sub whose figure looks like Kate Moss when they can have the curves of Cindy Crawford. Measuring your submissive for her corset (or his, in some instances), takes a great deal of precision, so I strongly suggest a very careful fitting before any purchase. While some prefer to leave this exacting process to a professional, many dominants (myself included) find that measuring a submissive for a corset can be a delightful task in and of itself.

Measuring to buy a corset isn't complicated. First, determine what it is you are looking for. Do you want something that will cover the breasts or leave them exposed? Do you plan to do waist training or just wear it occasionally?

Most people plan to wear their corsets only occasionally. Since they probably won't need a custom corset, measuring is simple. Measure your chest at the broadest part, be sure to include your waist and hips. The measurements don't have to be exact but should be close. You should also make a note if you are long- or short-waisted.

If you are planning to get a custom corset, you will need a few more measurements. Along with the chest, waist, and hip, you will need to measure the area under the breast around the ribs, the middle of the breast to the waist, the waist to the hip, and the length of your torso. Be sure to get the measurements from the front, back, and sides. The measurement, for instance, of the waist to the hip from the front will be different, in most cases, from the same measurement taken from the side or back.

If you have any unusual features, you will want to tell the salesperson as well. If you are disproportionately large- or small-busted, or have an unusual curvature of the spine, you will need to make this known to assure a good fit.

It is easier, and a lot more fun, to put on a corset and properly lace it with someone to help you, but it is also a task you can do yourself with relative ease. To put a corset on, first loosen the lacing in the back, and then fasten the front, usually with buckles, hooks, or a zipper. Then tighten the laces, working toward the middle from both the top and bottom, and tie the ends with a neat bow.

heels

I don't know who invented the high heel, but all women owe him a lot.

—MARILYN MONROE

No item you wear sends a clearer signal about who you are than your choice of footwear. One cannot imagine Elsa Klensch in anything less than the latest Prada pumps, just as Michael Jordan would seem like an athletic wanna-be if he played basketball wearing anything other than his signature Nikes.

The same case can be made for high heels, as they have a unique knack for making anyone who dares to wear them look sexier and command attention. Heels can have several effects on one's appearance, besides the obvious one of making you taller. They give the illusion of longer legs, smaller feet, higher buttocks, more prominent breasts, and better posture. As seen from behind, every step you take will give your backside a nice little shake, as well as a bit of a wobble in your leg.

With the resurgence in popularity of very high heels, there has been an increase in dire warnings from a phalanx of podiatrists and orthopedists about the dangers of these shoes. Among these concerns are an increase in lower back problems, bunions, and hammertoes, as well as a dangerous and unnatural stretching of the Achilles tendon. While such warnings should not be lightly dismissed, most of these problems can be ameliorated if you use your head before your feet. By using care in shopping; conditioning your feet, ankles, and legs; practicing a bit; and wearing a healthy mix of shoe heights and types, it is quite possible to walk in high heels comfortably for long periods of time without damaging your feet.

It is often difficult to make the adjustment to heels if your feet are not accustomed to them. If you have spent most of your life wearing flats, your feet are going to protest at being stuffed into five-inch heels. If your dominant insists on your being shod in stilettos, suggest an initial compromise: slightly lower heels, which will allow your feet some time to adjust to new heights. There are stunning shoes that can be found in mainstream shoe stores that have the fetish look, minus the risk of nosebleed. As an added bonus, you can wear them any time and not receive the looks you would get if you wore your stilettos to the office. Most people can begin by wearing a two-inch heel comfortably; all you need to do is gradually increase the height in half-inch increments.

High heels come in two basic styles: those without platforms, like the classic opera pump, and those with platforms, which I call Carmen Miranda shoes. You can calculate your ideal heel height by using your foot size as a base measurement. Simply measure your foot from the heel to the base of the toes and divide this measurement in half. The laws of physics dictate the higher the heel, the more pressure will be placed on the ball of your foot. Therefore, platforms that extend from the ball of your foot to the tips of your toes will help decrease this pressure because the wedge under your toes helps displace your weight more uniformly. For shoes with a platform base, you can generally add one inch of actual heel height.

When running out to Barneys or Saks for a new pair of heels, it is usually a good idea to get high heels that are at least half a size, or sometimes a whole size, larger than the shoes you usually wear. (Don't fret; remember, your feet will ultimately look smaller.) You will want this slightly larger size because your feet tend to swell as the day goes on, and the swelling will be exacerbated by a higher heel.

If you wish to move past starter stilettos, the proper exercises to increase the muscular strength in your feet and legs can be invaluable. (See "Just for Feet," page 178.)

walk this way

I can't see how anyone would object to a lady at the height of her beauty without any clothes on whatsoever . . . but, I would say it is even better with a pair of high heel shoes.

—VIVIENNE WESTWOOD

Adding several inches to your height will inevitably affect how you walk. Small, careful steps are the order of the day. Long, quick strides will only result in a short, hard trip to the floor.

When you are ready to make the move to sexy, dangerously-high heels, use every opportunity to wear them around the house before venturing out for an evening in them. Simply wearing heels while you are watching TV, writing out checks to your favorite charities, or even sleeping, will help your feet get accustomed to their new accoutrements.

Stilettos will cause your weight to be displaced differently than if you are barefooted or wearing flats. As you take your first steps, concentrate on keeping your weight centered over the middle of your feet as you are walking. Tuck in your derriere and lead from the hip, as if there were wires pulling you forward from there. This visualization will help you keep from walking bent over. Also, don't use your arms to balance; instead, practice walking with your hands held in the small of your back.

All these considerations and practice may seem like a lot of effort, but it is well worth it, as the appeal of the heel is irresistible.

what color is your perversion?

black

Unlike the fashion houses of Paris and Milan that change "in" colors with each new release of the Pantone color wheel, the one constant in the world of D/s is black. Black, especially in the case of a dominant, exudes a sense of power. It is also very slimming.

Black accentuates the shine on the rivets of a corset or the O-rings of your favorite collar. The sheen of a black latex outfit is an especially pleasing treat to the eye, while a pair of black leather gloves across the creamy skin of a submissive's derriere present an interesting contrast of both colors and textures. But you will never find the people you are looking for at a BDSM event by telling them, "I'll be the one in black," so I always urge my friends to expand their playtime palettes with some popular colors listed below.

red

Red is a color rife with sexual innuendo. It is the color of Valentine's Day, the traditional holiday of love, sex, and passion. Red catches our attention and then holds us an arm's length away. Female dominants will often have several items of red in their wardrobes, and they all know the allure of fiery red stilettos and the sensuality of plump lips lined in black and accentuated with searing red Chanel lipstick. Red stitching on the otherwise traditional plain black garb of a male dominant adds a sense of flair and style to the outfit, in the same way a bow tie breaks up some of the tedium of the tuxedo, a gentleman's version of the *robe de style*.

pink

Pink is a good color for both female and male submissives. It is feminine, yet still imbued with a touch of sexuality derived from its first cousin, red. Pink connotes a sense of naïveté, and it acquiesces to other, stronger colors, and, by extension, people.

white

White is the traditional sign of youth and innocence, so it is appropriate for submissives (even those whose idea of virginity is a new partner on Saturday night). There is also something terribly sexy about someone dressed in the pure white of a wedding gown performing wonderfully erotic acts.

blue

Show your elegance and affection by donning the most regal of all colors, blue. This color always complements black and keeps you from looking like Johnny Cash. Blue also exudes a sense of serenity, which a composed dom will maintain during even the most titillating of scenes.

bdsm glamour dos and don'ts

shaving

Shaved pubic hair is common for women who are into BDSM, especially submissives. Its popularity is based on aesthetics as well as practicality. Most dominants enjoy the exposed look of a well-groomed pubic area, and, of course, being shaved eliminates the potential embarrassment of shedding during intimate interaction.

While the prospect of pubic shaving may appear daunting at first, it is a simple (although time-consuming) process that is easily maintained and requires no more upkeep than shaving your legs.

Having your partner shave you can be a wonderfully erotic experience in and of itself. The following tips for shaving can be used by an individual or couple.

SHAVING FOR THE FIRST TIME

You will need:

- a small pair of scissors (one used to trim beards works well, as do embroidery scissors)
- a disposable razor (women's disposable razors with aloe strips are recommended)

- shaving cream (I like gels for sensitive skin)
- a small hand mirror with magnifier, especially if you are shaving yourself
- witch hazel

1. Trim as much hair as possible with the scissors. You will be amazed at how much hair can be removed this way and it will make the task of shaving infinitely easier. Trimming first will also keep you from going through two or three razors the first time.
2. Take a hot shower or a long, hot bath to initially soften the hair. Alternately, you can apply some warm, wet face cloths to the pubic area about five minutes before you begin shaving.
3. Liberally apply the shaving cream on the area you wish to shave. Let it sit there for at least a minute to allow it to soften the hair and the hair shaft. As you begin shaving, you may need to reapply some shaving cream.
4. Begin to shave by working from the outside in—that is, from your bikini line to your labia—making sure to rinse and clean the razor frequently. Remember that unlike the hair on your legs, pubic hair grows in all directions, so a diligent shaving in this delicate area should use strokes that go both with and against the grain. While it is common sense to use extra care when shaving both the inner and outer labia, this area is no more susceptible to shaving nicks than other parts of the body, so there is no need to fear an embarrassing trip to the emergency room.
5. Use the small hand mirror to help you see any hard-to-view areas. If you are shaving someone else, you can also

use the hand mirror to show your partner your handiwork.
6. After rinsing off, use witch hazel to help close your pores
   and prevent razor burn.

Note: *Never* use a depilatory like Neet or Nair on your
pubic hair, as that area is far too sensitive for such harsh
chemicals. If you want the shaved look, but have an unnatural fear of razors, you can try Magic Shave, a depilatory made
for African-American men. While many women have
reported using this product safely and effectively, *apply it first
on a small test area and wait for twenty-four hours to see if you
have any adverse reactions to it.*

Most people can get away with shaving every two or three
days, although your mileage may vary. The easiest way to do
this is in the shower after you have shampooed and condi-
tioned. By then, the stubble will have had a chance to soften.

If you want a very close shave, wait until your pubic area
is easily observed as being stubbly (usually three or four days
after your last shave) and use a razor you have already used
once or twice.

makeup

Dramatic makeup with deep colors, especially black and
red, is always an appropriate choice for D/s cosmetics. While
anyone can pile on tons of black eye shadow and mascara, here
are a couple of suggestions to keep you ahead of the pack.

Reverse French Manicure: A reverse French manicure is
a simple, elegant attention-getter. Just ask your manicurist
for black nails with white tips. No need to feel odd about it;
she has gotten far stranger requests.

Black lipstick: What could be better for a night in the dungeon? To keep it on, first apply a layer of lipstick, blot, then apply a layer of black eye shadow. Repeat twice.

seven steps to sexy

Just like planning for a typical evening when haute couture is de rigueur, you must employ the same amount of detail and planning for a night in the realm of S & M.

1. Has your dominant ordered something in particular?
   If yes, skip to Step 5.
   If no, continue to Step 2.
2. Is there a particular theme?
   If yes, skip to Step 5.
   If no, continue to Step 2.
3. Will you be at:
   a) a private home other than your own, or
   b) your own home or a club?
   If (a), proceed to Step 4.
   If (b), skip to Step 5.
4. If you have already been a guest at your host's home, carefully consider the design and decor so as to avoid clashing with your surroundings. (You don't want to be dressed as a Renaissance serving wench in a home with a strong Lichtenstein influence.) Proceed to Step 5.
5. Do a thorough review of your closets, armoires, trunks, and bureaus before deciding if a shopping expedition is necessary. Remember, you can get extra life out of your clothing by being a careful accessory consumer.
   If shopping is required, proceed to Step 6.
   If no shopping is required, skip to Step 7.

6. If shopping is required, stop for a minute before your call to book an appointment at your favorite fetish emporium. If your party has an Elizabethan or Gothic theme, consider some of the wonderful items you can find at a Renaissance festival. Or scout out local vintage and consignment shops, for it is in places like this where you can often find unusual items at great prices. Proceed to Step 7.

7. Carefully examine the outfit you have selected. Make sure there are no runs in your stockings, your heels are free of scuff marks, and all your satins, leathers, and synthetics are shiny.

suggestions for other occasions

the bdsm organization meeting

Most people who attend meetings of D/s organizations, such as New York City's Eulenspiegel Society, are arriving directly from work. There are a lot of men in tailored pants who have exchanged their white button-down shirt for a black T-shirt, while women will tend to dress conservatively while also demurely displaying their best assets. If you are feeling adventurous, find out what the evening's topic is and dress accordingly: a catsuit for bondage; for back-to-school night, a white blouse with a Peter Pan collar, short pleated skirt, lacy anklets, and patent leather Mary Janes.

bdsm clubs

Casual dress is also acceptable for public BDSM clubs, but this is more the rule for men than for women. These clubs are often viewed as where you go to strut your stuff. At the very least, a submissive woman with an escort should always wear La Perla panties (in case the opportunity to play presents itself), a nice collar, one item of leather clothing, and high heels with a minimum heel height of four inches. Dominant women tend to dress to the nines on all occasions (you will notice that many of the professionals look like Xena the Warrior Princess on a good day). No woman attending a BDSM club or party should leave her house before copiously apply searing red lipstick. (And be sure to have a tube in your purse—you can't always count on a transvestite being in the ladies' room to bail you out.)

bdsm parties

Parties, sponsored either by a club or by a private host, are where you will want to wear your nicest things, because everyone will be doing likewise. Whatever makes you feel the sexiest—or pleases your dominant the most—is in order, because this is the perfect time to act out your clothing fantasies. If you have always wanted to try body paint, or longed for an opportunity for you and your dominant to dress as Sweet Gwen and Sir D'Arcy, respectively, here's your chance.

With a virtually endless choice of colors, fabrics, and designers to chose from, you should have no problem creating a fabulous fetish wardrobe that will be an embodiment of your personality and sense of style.

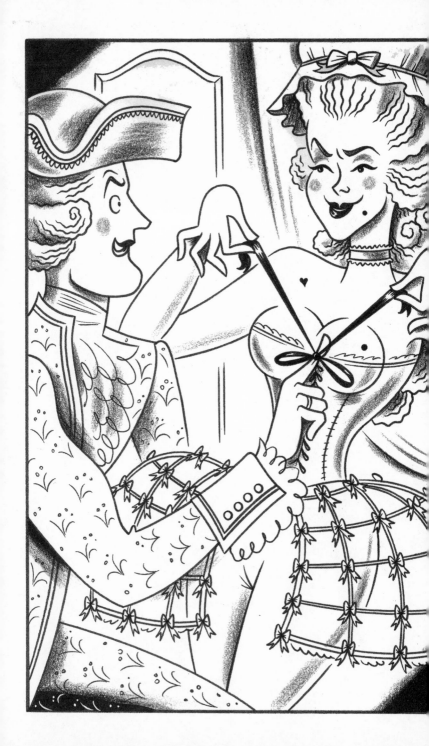

- 4 -

ON BEING
KNOTTY

practical ropework for impractical situations

*No cord or cable can draw so forcibly, or bind so fast,
as love can do with a single thread.*
—ROBERT BURTON

To paraphrase La Rochefoucauld, bondage "lessens halfhearted passions, and increases great ones, as the wind puts out the candle, yet stirs up the coals." This physical act of your lover relinquishing his or her personal power to you is at the very core of the D/s forbidden fruit, and more simply, one huge turn-on for many. Chances are if you have one kink in your straight rope, this is it, whether it was because you were held down helplessly and tickled by your older brother's cute friends or you just identified with all those hapless heroines getting trussed and displayed on Saturday morning action dramas.

Restraint is the basis of good manners, and nowhere else but in a BDSM relationship does this statement have such literal simplicity. While there are specialty shops and skilled craftsmen galore selling all manner of manacles, a working knowledge of rope and knots is a basic bedroom skill one needs not only to develop, but—pardon the expression— master. The look in his eye when you whip out a perfect bowline without looking, fumbling, or breaking a nail will show that you have cemented his attention faster than Krazy Glue, and you both will definitely get all wrapped up in lovemaking —with strings attached.

Knots and rope bondage have been obsessions of mine since childhood. I can remember being around eight or nine, curled up on the Berber carpet in front of the sitting room's red granite fireplace with the *Boy Scout Fieldbook*, fascinated by even the Tenderfoot knot work. Later, I matriculated to the *Bluejackets Manual*, handbook of the U.S. Navy. While marlinespike seamanship is not necessary for your binder primer, it is as important to know what knot is proper for which occasion as it is to know how to match a purse with shoes. A working knowledge of knots is a handy crossover skill, one for which you will find more everyday use than, say, whip cracking. Your gift-wrapping skills will be indispensable at holidays. But before we get into the twists and ties of the friendly confines, let's define some trussing terms.

theory of bondgitivity

I cleave sexual bondage into two schools of thought. One is binding your lover simply to capture, immobilize, and have your way with him. The second division is bondage as a living human art form, literally bondage for art's sake. Needless to say, this way of thinking is a bit more advanced. But even if you are just into bow-tying your beau, you want to look like you know what you are doing.

At the risk of sounding like some corseted insurance agent, two concepts reign supreme in the restraint of one's submissive: safety and security. Your slave for the evening will be a helpless, well-wrapped package whose life or limbs are never at risk; comfortable, yet knowing that the least amount of struggle will increase discomfort and immobility.

Artistically trussing your treasure allows for limitless possibilities of self-expression, which can improve the ambience of even the most routine bondage situations. When considering a new bondage opportunity, I carefully assess what kind of statement my choice of bonds will make. Will this be a basic training session? An elaborate fantasy scene? Should my submissive feel cherished or humiliated? Does the slave consider bondage punishment or a special treat? What time of day or night will we be playing? Are there seasonal or special personal symbolic themes that can be incorporated?

constriction vs. extension

In the same way that bondage can be divided into two schools of thought, there are again two broad strokes of bondage styles. These opposite styles are drawing the limbs apart and holding the limbs together—or, put more succinctly, *constriction* and *extension*. There is endless variety in each of these disciplines. As a rule, the limbs must be drawn apart if you require your slave to be open and exposed for your (or his) pleasure. Conversely, the limbs should be tied together, once again in numerous ways, for more of a punishment or kidnap feel, or bondage for art's sake. For example, the arms bound tightly from behind can enhance the bosom of a female sub as no Wonderbra can.

The pinioning of the limbs in constriction bondage is much less of an exposition for the submissive than in extension bondage, and consequently has a much more intimate appeal. I often think of constriction bondage as "hugging by proxy." The ultimate goal in constriction bondage—its Holy Grail—is the meeting of the elbows behind the back. Of course, not everyone's anatomy allows this. For those that do not, there are several knots and arrangements of knots that will help gain enough mechanical advantage to coax the limbs as close as possible.

A "trucker's hitch" will work for this. Novices may find it helpful to think of this as blocks and tackles made out of loops of rope. You can also use an "Alpine Butterfly," which even sounds like a sexual position, above each elbow to form loops that can be cinched tight with another piece of rope. For those of you with more *dinero* than dexterity, a calfskin arm binder, also known as a single glove, will allow you to accomplish this behind-the-back artistry in a more comfortable fashion. These are, however, hard to explain if they happen to fall out of your closet at an inopportune time.

Once the elbows are secured, tying the wrists often becomes unnecessary, but it is still not altogether useless. Here you can ad lib and keep the hands straight out from the elbows behind the back or wrapped around in front towards the tummy. Another interesting elbow tie is with the elbow swung forward and above the head and tied as closely as possible. The wrists are then bound together and tethered to a crotch rope from behind. A word of caution, however; even advanced "tie-ees" cannot last long with the arms bound so severely, so do not keep your sub in this position for too long. Also, be extremely careful not to burn the skin by excitedly pulling the bulk of the rope against a soft-tissue body part. After a few minutes, it is time to untie and try new positions (it helps the musculature to alternate constriction bondage with extension bondage) and a little rubdown on the limbs of your sub is certain to increase his devotion to you. Plus, keep in mind that if the sensations are more painful than pleasing, the chances of bondage becoming a regular feature of your lovemaking are diminished.

In extension bondage, like the classic "spread eagle" position, the foremost thing to keep in mind is to position the knots well away from the fingers. This enables you to tie quick-release knots, which can save time and trouble. Facedown or faceup on the bed or coffee table, spread and bent over the back of a chair, or even tied against a door are all positions that lend themselves to extension bondage.

Using fetish clothing on the extremities, such as gloves and spike-heel shoes, can add to the helplessness of the bottom by taking away dexterity. Special bondage clothing, such as mitts and the aforementioned arm binder, are useful and have their place, but are not necessary.

the dope on rope

Before tying your first knot, you must have something to tie it with, and the most classic bondage accoutrement of all is rope. Rope is made from a myriad of natural and man-made fibers, and can be either laid (three strands twisted together) or woven. Different materials are used for different applications, but almost any rope can be used to truss up a lover. Among the naturals are hemp, sisal, manila, and cotton. The first three, especially sisal, leave little irritating hairs behind (like having one more shedding pet). They are rough to the touch (yours and your victim's) and lend sort of a hardened, butch look to your work.

Cotton, on the other hand, has qualities making it unfit for most industrial applications, but almost perfect for human bondage. While not as strong as other natural and synthetic rope, it is plenty strong to hold down a man. An added bonus is that it is soft to the touch, which really cuts down on the abrasion factor. The laid variety is very soft and decorative, and even the woven stuff, like sash cord, has the benefit of being some of the cheapest rope on the market. You can use yards of it and not worry about making the payment on the Porsche. Far and away the most comfortable cotton rope I have ever used is special magician's rope, 3/8-inch diameter woven around a hollow core. And yes, you can buy it at magic specialty stores.

The synthetics are easier to find these days, and will certainly do the job of trussing your loved one. Besides the original synthetic, nylon, there are polyester and several types of polypropylene. Nylon is stretchy, relatively cheap, and available in a variety of diameters. Some of the polypropylene ropes are not "bedroom quality," so look for "filibrated" or "staple-spun" polypropylene. These have the aesthetic appeal of natural rope and a texture the hand can easily grip.

Mountaineering rope, with its fine braided sheath and twisted core, is very luxurious and functional, but because of its quality controls it is very expensive. Unless it is well worn (thus, ironically, unfit for mountain climbing) it is too stiff and unmanageable to work well for small knots. But, on the plus side, it does come in a variety of designer colors that can match any decor or outfit, if you are that much of a slave to fashion. And mountaineering rope is simply a must when you have your slave costumed in lederhosen.

whips are not just for tushes

Sooner or later you're going to have to cut your rope into usable lengths. (I like to keep 7/16-inch diameter rope in ten- and twenty-foot sections.) Whether braided or twisted, the ends will unravel when you cut it if you don't do something. This "something" is called "whipping," but it is not as much fun as it sounds. There are several wimpy ways to do it: wrapping with electrical tape, dipping in liquid latex or glue, or using a cigarette lighter (synthetics only). For the really inspired, heat-shrink tubing, available at electronic stores and melted with a dryer that looks like a hair dryer on steroids, will do a neat job on the ends. The quickest way is cutting with a "hot knife" that melts as it slices (expensive synthetic mountaineering rope is cut this way).

But the idea is to make you an accomplished domme, and the most impressive way to keep from coming unraveled at the end of your rope is to, with apologies to Devo, whip it good. Once again there are several styles of whipping, but one of the easiest is called American whipping.

American Whipping

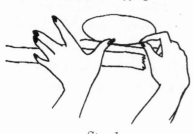

Step 1

Lay a length of thread (waxed sail twine works best) parallel to the rope near the rope's end, and form an overhand loop by turning the ends of the thread so they are parallel with the rope and extending out in opposite directions. With your left thumb, hold the point of the loop at which the two ends cross against the rope. With your right hand, grab the right side of the loop at about three o' clock and begin to neatly wind the thread around and around the end of the rope (and the thread ends lying against it) until you run out of the original loop that was formed. Then pull on the two ends of the thread sticking out from under the coils (in opposite directions) until all the

American Whipping (cont'd.)

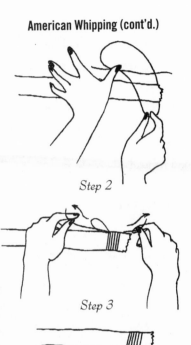

Step 2

Step 3

Step 4

slack is taken out of the thread loop and the whipping is tight. Trim the ends that stick out of the coils with a knife or scissors. Your whipping should be as long as the rope is thick.

you are kinky, your rope is not

As a domme, you should be meticulously neat, and neatness in storing your rope supplies means coiling. This doesn't mean extra work for you, but you should know how it is done to teach your submissives to do it correctly. There is a natural twist to three-strand laid rope when it is first uncoiled.

S-laid rope has a counterclockwise twist; Z-laid rope has a clockwise twist. Which is which? Look at the rope lying flat. Do the strands run in a / (Z) or \ (S) pattern? If you can remember to follow that twist when you or subbie-boy coils the rope, it will be less of a bird's nest. Lay the coils one by one in your flat palm and restore the twist by turning the rope just so with your thumb and forefinger. It is considered bad rope etiquette to wind it around your elbow and hand like a vacuum-cleaner electrical cord. In fact, it is bad vacuum-cord etiquette, too.

to have and have knot

The icing on the bondage cake is the knot, trussing's raison d'être. These simple means to an end may confuse a novice dominant, but knots are a basic and easily mastered bondage skill. A few knots are all one needs to know, and learning to tie and untie them quickly can save not only embarrassment, but perhaps life or limb.

Knots fall into three categories: *bends,* or knots for joining two ropes or two ends of a rope together; knots for forming a loop in the end or middle of a rope; and knots for attaching the end of a rope to something else, such as a bedpost or an ankle.

Some other tying terms will help in the step-by-step explanation of how to fashion these knots. The *running* end of the rope is the part closest to the end that you are using to tie the knot. The *standing* end is the stationary or inactive part the running end is tied around. A *bight* is a rope bent back on itself, and a *loop* is a circle formed in the rope crossing the standing part. If it is an *underhand* loop, the running end is under the standing end; if it is *overhand,* the running end is over the standing part. (Some knot-headed authorities call these loops *crossing turns,* meaning that the running end has crossed the standing end, but I am the domme here and we will use my definitions.)

One other thing: many people can follow directions about the standing ends, running ends, and loops, but end up with just an embarrassing jumble of cord when completed because they don't pull on the right parts when tightening the finished product. You may have it tied correctly and then blow the finish when you go to cinch it. Try to keep a picture of the knot in your mind when you are learning a new knot. Practice makes perverts.

knots ready for prime tying

The square or reef knot, while not as dependable as its reputation would have us believe, and the "slipped" variation of the square knot, are good starts for joining the two ends of the same piece of rope together. The bowline is the unslippable choice for putting a loop in the end of a rope. A clove hitch is a great choice for attaching a rope to cylindrical objects, as is the two half hitches. You can use both by finishing a clove hitch with two half hitches for an even more secure tie.

Only a bit more challenging is the taut-line hitch. This knot will hold its place wherever it is positioned along the standing end of a tightened line. This feature allows a dominant to easily adjust the length of any rope, like the ones used to hold your hands to the headboard. If you need to join two different pieces of rope together, of the same or different diameters, the best choice is the sheet bend. The easiest knot, the overhand, and its relative, the figure-eight knot, are also useful to know. These can be used at the end of your rope, and are useful for keeping the end from slipping through an O-ring you may have conveniently positioned near your bed. They can also be used in series along a length of cord for a version of the "nine knots of love," but that is another topic in itself.

None of these knots is particularly difficult to tie. Tying an impossible knot is not the secret to rendering your partner helpless; the key is to put a simple knot out of his reach. Proper placement makes all the difference.

a slippery situation

Bondage being the kind of naughty fun it is, it seems as though there is always a reason to get untied in a hurry. Like your mother showing up for tea, or noticing fire engines screeching to a halt outside your hotel window. Because of this, it is essential to tie your knots "slipped" (think of a single bow on your shoestring). This is easily done by making a "bend" in your running end and slipping it through the last part of your knot (instead of the actual end of the rope) when finishing your knot. (See the slipped square knot on p. 75)

where the strings are attached

On the subject of placement, there must be some anatomical consideration and some engineering common sense given to where on the body to attach the bindings. It goes without saying that the feet should be tied to keep a slave in place, and the hands should be restrained to prevent escape. In constriction bondage, I use the simple and time-tested three wraps and two fraps around the ankles, above and sometimes below the knees, and, of course, the wrists (not too tight; you must not cut off circulation). A wrap is perpendicular to the limbs, while a frap is parallel and between the limbs. Sometimes, if you have a particularly Houdini-esque partner, you can up the number of wraps. There has been much discussion about whether ankles and wrists should be tied crossed or uncrossed, but I believe there is a time and place for both. Certainly immobility is heightened by crossing the limbs, but sometimes the sub as an objet d'art calls for the streamlined look that uncrossing lends.

time and tied
wait for none

Taking a long time to tie up your partner can spoil an otherwise hot mood. A way to cut down on the tying time is to employ the Japanese style of lashing, where the rope is doubled, and the two running ends pass through the bight formed in the middle of the rope. An added benefit is this allows you to keep longer pieces of rope that come in handy when used in the normal fashion for upper arms, thighs, and chests of larger partners, as well as chair ties and the like. Japanese square-lashing works well on crossed ankles and wrists. The middle of the rope is hooked over, say, one ankle, and the two running ends of the rope cross over the other ankle and continue wrapping, leaving enough to change direction for the fraps and the final knot. The Japanese are also famous for their complicated diamond-hitch style of tying limbs and trunks, which is something that really has to be seen to be appreciated.

gender benders

While it is obvious that the hands and feet—and sometimes knees and elbows—need to be made fast in order to render a sub immobile, some thought should be given to other, more tender parts of the anatomy. A crotch rope, literally a binding of the lower part of the trunk, is a wonderful place to secure the ankles and the hands in a bow tie, either in front or back (the name most commonly used when the feet are tied to the hands behind the back is a *hog-tie,* but I think *bow tie* is a prettier name and more descriptive of the position). Any struggle by the slave pulls on the rope around this tender region, and exerts an exquisitely pleasurable-to-painful pressure that quickly extinguishes any notion of escape. The effect can be heightened with the addition of some well-placed overhand or figure-eight knots, especially in the *placa d'anus* or mound of Venus.

the breast is yet to come

Another favorite tender target on female submissives is the breasts. Breast bondage presents some challenges, but it can be an, ahem, uplifting experience for the master and certainly for the female slave. Unlike hands, breasts cannot untie themselves, and unlike feet, they are not going anywhere, so to bind them is one more extension of the tying tableau of artful bondage. While wrists and ankles don't vary much in their respective diameter among persons, breasts come in a varied array of sizes. How bosoms are to be tied depends on how much one has to work with. This is a good place to use a clove hitch, constricting the breast and swelling the area of the aureole and nipple for increased sensitivity. *Be very careful not to tie too tight or leave so long as to cause tissue damage.* After tying, the only thing needed is a feather or clamp, depending on your mood.

Larger breasts can be tied, with apologies to Playtex, in a "cross-your-heart" pattern, using the shoulders in much the same way as bra straps, with the knots in the back, out of the

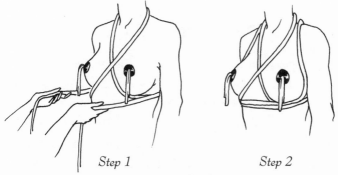

Step 1   *Step 2*

Breast Bondage

way. Start with the center of a ten- to twenty-foot length of rope on the back of the neck of your slave. Cross the running ends in front of the chest between the breasts in an X pattern and then under the armpits. Continue behind the middle of the back, crossing the running ends around the trunk and back around in front below the breasts and up between them, again in an X pattern.

It helps to have your submissive standing and bending over, which makes the breasts hang, and thus makes them easier to tie. Loop the running ends again around the back of the neck, cross again between the breasts and under the armpits, and finish with a slipped square knot behind the middle of the back. If you put one extra twist on the first overhand knot of the square knot, it will help hold the knot in place (as it would when you ask someone to do it with a finger while tying a bow) while you finish the second, and finishing, overhand knot. This variation of a square knot has its own name, the "surgeon's knot" (thank you, doctor). A rope brassiere such as this, like the crotch rope, makes an excellent anchor point for securing the limbs.

ty hardon

Of course, men have their own special protrusions that lend themselves to bondage. The male genitalia gives two other points of contact for the smaller diameters of rope and ribbon. Especially enjoyable is the Grecian Sandal wound up around the erect—and bound to stay that way—male member. This works like a cock ring, but, again, *be especially careful not to tie the knots too tightly, and always use a slipknot in*

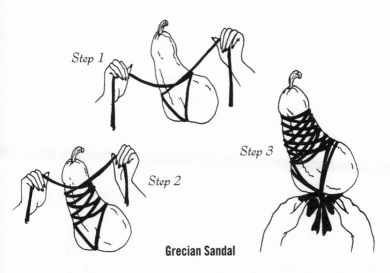

Step 1

Step 2

Step 3

Grecian Sandal

this area. Start from the base of the penis, including the testicles, with a small-diameter rope. Wind upward to the base of the head, then wind back down, finishing with a slipped square knot at the base of the testicles (or a full bow if you are feeling particularly decorative).

war-ning! dan-ger, will rope-inson!

I don't consider any of my readers idiots, but I must put this caveat in the text. *Do* exercise extreme caution when it comes to putting people into bondage. *Don't* use a person's neck for a lash point. *Do* check for discoloration or swelling on a tied limb. *Don't* tie a knot that can't be easily untied, and *quickly. Do* have a safe word that lets a domme know when enough is enough, and when the sub says "enough," untie *immediately. Don't* use rope that is too small in diameter and can cut into flesh. *Do* loosen frequently. *Don't* use baling wire. *Do* use slipknots. *Don't* leave the room when a person is gagged. *Do* pay very careful attention to your slave. *Don't* let him *think* you are paying attention to him (as that would spoil the mood). And by all means, *don't* leave this book where your priest, pastor, or rabbi can find it. Let him buy his own copy.

d/tails: enders, benders, hitches, and loops

the overhand knot

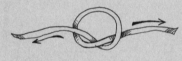

Overhand Knot

This is the simplest of all knots, and the building block or first step of many others. Once tied and pulled tight, though, it can be difficult to untie. 1) With the running end of your rope, make a loop around the standing end. 2) Pass the running end through the loop. 3) Pull tight. So simple.

the figure-eight knot

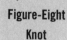

Figure-Eight Knot

This one actually looks like it sounds (a square knot certainly isn't square). It is used in the same situations as an overhand knot, but it's a little bulkier, which can be a good thing if it is rubbing up against anything sensitive. And it is easier to untie, which is always a good thing. 1) Make an overhand loop over the standing part of your rope. 2) Reverse the direction of the running end by crossing it over the standing end, making an underhand loop. 3) Pull the running end back through the original loop. If you have done this one right, it will look like a cross between the numeral eight and a dollar sign.

the square knot or reef knot

This most popular of knots, the most common of "bends," is actually a big impostor, because of its tendency to "capsize," or collapse and come untied. It was originally invented to keep sails tied up, or reefed, not a particularly critical application. It should never be used to join two ropes together in a life-threatening situation (like mountain climbing). But, for the purposes of bondage, it does work okay and is a very symmetrical and beautiful knot. And it is very easy to untie, especially "slipped" (more about this later). 1) Take the two running ends of a piece of rope and make an overhand knot, with the right end over

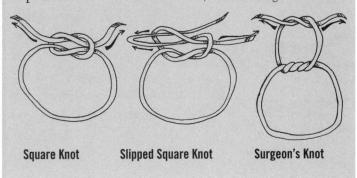

Square Knot   **Slipped Square Knot**   **Surgeon's Knot**

the left. 2) Now make another, with the left end over the right. 3) Pull tight. If you fail to do this correctly, you will end up with a granny knot. (Grannies are not bad knots, they just have a bad reputation because they are hard to untie. Which can be good if you are in a serious situation. If you are tying up your girlfriend—slipped square knots. If you are tying up the intruder you just coldcocked in your kitchen—granny knots and then some.)

To make a slipped square knot, make a bight on one of the running ends during step two. If you make a bight on both running ends, you will have a bow knot, also known as a shoelace knot. If you put an extra twist on the overhand knot in step one, you will have what is known as a surgeon's knot, which has the advantage of staying in place better (like asking someone to hold the knot with a finger) while you finish steps two and three.

the sheet bend

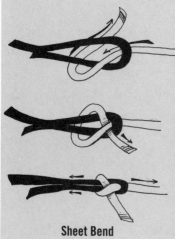

Sheet Bend

The square knot, described above, is often misused to join two different ropes together. The sheet bend is actually the preferred knot for this task. It will not collapse as easily as the square knot, is easy to tie and untie, and has the added advantage of being able to join ropes of different diameters together. 1) Make a bight on the end of the rope with the larger diameter (of course, the ropes can also be the same diameter). 2) Take the running end of the smaller rope, come up from under the bight on the larger rope, loop around and back under the standing part of the smaller rope without going back through the bight (which would be a square knot). For extra security, you can loop twice around the top of the bight before you tuck under the standing end. This is called a *double* sheet bend.

the two half hitches

The two half hitches is a great choice for securing a rope to a ring, a pole, or a bedpost. 1) Take your running end and pass it around the post or through the ring. 2) Then take the running end of the rope and tie a overhand knot (the "first" half hitch) around the standing part of

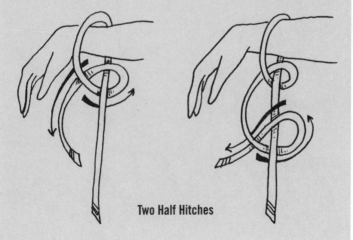

Two Half Hitches

the rope, but do not pull it tight. 3) With the running end, go around the standing part of the rope again in the same direction, bringing your running end between the two loops formed round the standing part of the rope. 4) Pull on both the standing end and the running end to pull tight. I don't know why this knot isn't called "The Full Hitch," since it is made of two halves, but it is not, so don't go there. You can improve its holding power substantially by passing a *round turn,* or extra wrap, around the post or ring before tying this knot.

the clove hitch

One of the best choices while tying a rope around a cylindrical object, the clove hitch is a model of simplicity in tying and untying. (It too, is made of two half hitches.) It

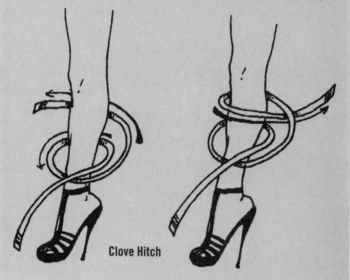

Clove Hitch

is very strong because the rope only wraps in one direction. 1) Wrap the running end of your rope around a post or pole. 2) Cross the running end of the rope over the standing part. 3) Take the running end and make a second turn around the pole in the same direction. 4) Pull the running end under the second turn and pull taut. There is a quicker, really cool domme trick to tying one of these if the top of your bedpost is accessible. 1) Holding the rope in your two hands, first make an overhand loop with your right hand over the standing part of the rope in your left hand and put your left thumb over it to hold it in place. 2) Repeat this procedure, making a second overhand loop and place it underneath the first loop. 3) Drop the whole rig over the open end of the pole and pull tight with both hands. With a little practice you can do this in less than a second and really strike delicious awe in your slave.

the taut-line hitch

This knot is unusual in that it will adjust to itself— that is, the knot will slide and hold along the tight, standing part of the rope. Its main use is securing tent guylines to stakes. With a little imagination, you can substitute a slave pup for a pup tent. It is tied much like the two half hitches, with an extra turn before you make the final hitch (I know, why isn't it called three half hitches?). 1) Bring the running end of your rope around the pole (or stake) and make one loop around the standing part of your rope. 2) Make one more loop, going toward the pole.

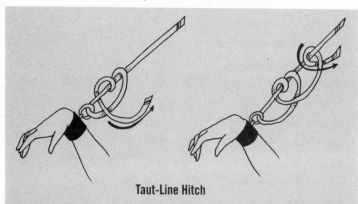

Taut-Line Hitch

3) Make a third loop around your standing end by bringing your running end back around over both loops toward the running end. 4) Pull the running end through on the inside of the last loop formed. 5) Tighten by sliding the knot up and down the standing end.

the bowline

The bowline is the Domme of the loops; it holds well and is easy to tie and untie. 1) Make a small overhand loop on the standing part of your rope after leaving a generous supply of running end (this will eventually be the size of your loop). 2) Take the tip of the running end, and from underneath go through the small loop you have made, up around the standing part, and then back into the loop. (This is the famous "rabbit" who comes out from his hole, runs around the tree, and goes back in the hole. Corny, but thousands have learned to tie this knot with that description.) 3) Hold on to the standing part above the loop and the running end that is just peeking

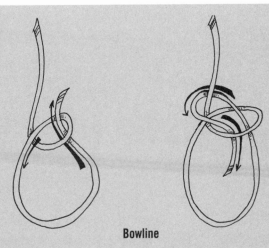

Bowline

underneath through the loop and pull tight. If you put the other end of the rope through the bowline you have just tied, you have a "running bowline," which can pull tight (think of a lariat loop, although this is not the knot used to tie lariats).

the alpine butterfly

You have to love the name of this knot. I keep seeing Heidi on her back with her legs in the air on some ledge on Mont Blanc. This is one of the best ways to put a nonslippable loop in the middle of a rope. 1) With the palm of your left hand open and facing you, take the middle of your rope and wrap it loosely around your left hand,

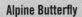

Alpine Butterfly

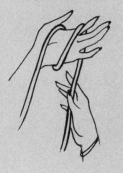

Alpine Butterfly (cont'd.)

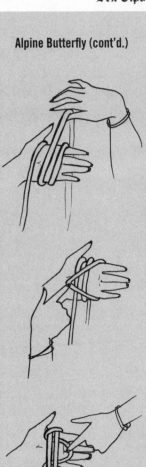

going from the bottom of your palm to the top. 2) Wrap another loop, close to the fingers of your left hand. 3) Wrap a third loop, this time going between the other two loops you have made on your hand. 4) Then, with your right hand, pull on the loop closest to the fingers of your left hand (the second loop you made) and bring it over the other two loops and then underneath all three. 5) Pull tight and you will have a nice loop. A pair of these tied in a rope above the elbows will allow you to cinch the arms down very tightly. A more boring application is tightening down loads, such as a deer, to the roof rack of your car. Or combine both skills and tie your lover boy to the roof of your car. Look, a one-point buck! Good hunting.

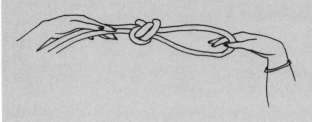

the trucker's hitch

The trucker's hitch is actually a combination of knots that acts like a simple block and tackle to get a line tighter than Rosie Perez's capri pants. 1) On one end of your rope is a loop knot, such as a bowline (if you are tying to the middle, use the alpine butterfly). 2) With

Trucker's Hitch

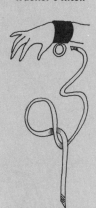

plenty of slack on the running end of the rope, form an overhand loop, and twist it one more time. 3) Then pass a bight of the running end through the loop just formed. 4) Take the running end and pass through your original bowline or butterfly. 5) Bring the running end back down through the bight that is peeking through the loop. 6) Cinch tight, and finish with two half hitches. This is good on the D-rings of manacles above the elbows, too.

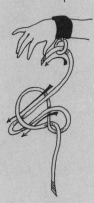

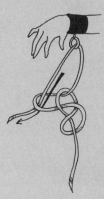

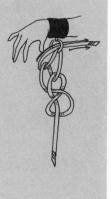

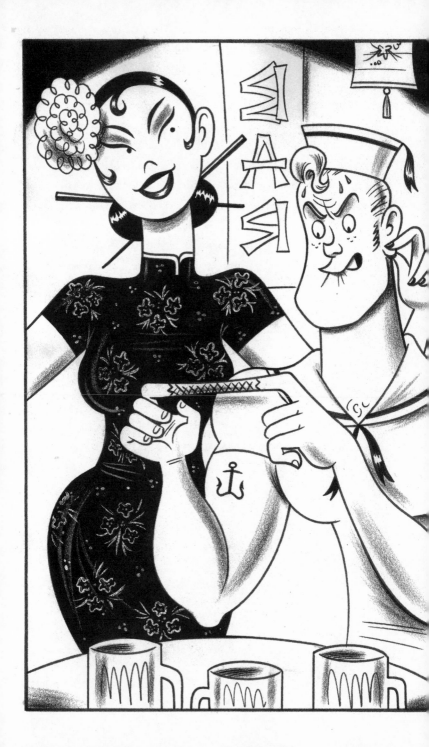

- 5 -

BONDAGE 201

other ties that bind

Now that you have had a chance to learn the ropes, it is time to think beyond just tying up your partner and enter a whole new world of bondage convenience. For although a knowledge of ropework is an excellent basic skill to have, it is not necessary to use it exclusively. Think of it as learning Latin, a discipline that lays a foundation for further study. There are many other contraptions of confinement, some designed for the job and some adapted from other purposes. An introduction to these can save time on the tying, allowing more time for other, less restrictive endeavors.

cuff links

Handcuffs are probably the most widely known of the metal restraining devices. Unless you know escape-artist tricks of the trade (and many of their "tricks" are as simple as hiding a key or having a secret latch) these can be nearly impossible to get out of, even with a hacksaw. Handcuffs have probably caused more embarrassment than any other bondage accessory, owing to the Murphy's law that states that keys are almost always lost or misplaced.

On the other hand, no accoutrement says "good cop/bad cop" better than professional handcuffs. It says you mean business. It says you are mean. Unless your sub has large limbs, they can also be used on ankles and in multiple combinations for very harsh and uncomfortable bow ties. I always keep a couple of sets in my domme box, for even if I do not use them often, they simply look so evil and ready to use.

They are also a collectible: while certainly not as cuddly as Beanie Babies, there is a black (and blue) market for vintage manacles, such as the English Darby cuffs and Tower cuffs. Usually, handcuffs are connected with a chain, but there do exist cuffs with rigid metal bars and others with single hinges. There are websites where you can pick up old iron ones or new aluminum ones. A good place to start, with links to several more sites, is Yossie's Handcuff Collection at www.blacksteel.com.

On the downside, handcuffs hurt—and not necessarily in a good way—so proceed with extreme caution. They can chafe, they can pinch when being clasped on, they can cause bruises, and—if they are too tight—they can cut off the circulation to the hands and feet. They can also scar the Chippendale. They were designed for police, who probably don't have a lot of playtime fun with bondage (although I could be wrong about this). If you plan to play this heavy, as always, be extremely careful. Never clasp handcuffs on too tight—always make sure there is at least a little finger's width between the cuff and the wrist's radial protrusion. Constantly look for any discoloration of the attached extremity.

And write this next tip down: *Have spare keys*. More than one set. If you are the submissive, have your own set. If you are a domme, have an extra set hidden where only *you* know, just in case the tables are turned, Heaven forbid.

thumbs up

If space in your domme box is limited, then this is the minimanacle you need—thumbcuffs. Ingeniously small, inscrutably efficient, they lock between the first and second joints of the thumb, or they can also be used on the big toes. It is a maddening feeling to be so lightly, yet so helplessly, restrained. Diminutive size does not mean diminutive performance, so all of the key precautions listed above apply.

a better fetter

More comfortable than metal handcuffs are leather manacles. These cuffs are adjustable and, with the addition of little luggage-style padlocks, lockable. They also look very hot. Some are even lined with fur and come in a variety of widths for extra comfort. Leather manacles on your slave allow for tying, untying, and retying into various positions quickly and relatively effortlessly. Special suspension cuffs, *the only way* I recommend full feet-off-the-floor suspension, have a device to prevent wrist stress, and are recommended if your "swinger" has carpal tunnel syndrome or the like. What also works well with these are double-spring clasps, available from any hardware store. You can combine these with chain, metal O-rings, and even rope.

If you don't want to make a special trip to the bondage store, a wonderful substitute are the D-ringed cuffs used on a cable-crossover exercise machine. A perfect choice, they are extrasturdy to handle the strain of all those weight plates. They are made in leather, fleece-lined, and adjustable with a buckle. They also come in nylon, with infinitely adjustable and very innocent looking Velcro straps. (While we are on the subject, the cable-crossover machine itself is a great accessory for extension bondage. You can have your pet go from one workout to another.)

go ahead, collar, you're on the line

Speaking of pets, nothing completes a leather manacle ensemble like a collar around the neck of your slave. Whether actually made for a large dog or a human, whether studded or all metal, or even the tall "posture" variety, collars more than anything else are the symbol of D/s servitude. The collar is to a BDSM relationship what the wedding band is to a marriage, although subs aren't given a jeweled "engagement choker" as a prelude to the real thing. In D/s lingo, a sub would say she is "collared" (in a relationship and not looking) or "uncollared" (single and available). Sometimes, though, the collar is just a fashion statement, sometimes even worn by a top. I own several. One of my favorites, a gift from a submissive who owned a jewelry store, is a brushed sterling silver hinge-and-clasp model. I am hoping for matching handcuff earrings soon.

Collars are more than symbolic, however. With their attached rings, they are a relatively safe way to use the neck in bondage, as long as it is not used to suspend the slave (I think the technical term for this is *hanging* and the legal term is *homicide*—so DON'T do it!). The same precautions for tightness are even more critical around the neck than with other extremities. The rings on your slave's collar also share the same use as those on your Doberman's, a place to anchor the leash. Sit! Heel! Beg! Good boy.

chaining training

Chains are so much a symbol of the bondage experience that when paired with whips, as in "whips and chains," the phrase is shorthand for the entire D/s lifestyle. Chain is a heavier statement, both figuratively and literally, than rope. Some submissives are really into the weight of the chain wrapped tightly around the body (more Jacob Marley than Bob, who would of course be done up in hemp). Chains can also be clasped or locked to the above-mentioned handcuffs and manacles. Freezing the chain first is fun and a guaranteed eye-opener for your chilled consort.

high-priced spread

A novel way to achieve extension bondage is with spreader bars pushing the limbs out as opposed to rope tethers pulling the limbs out. These should have rings or holes at the end to tie or clasp the ankles and wrists so they are far apart. Some more costly bars have manacles built into the ends; some even have collars built in the center. Escape from these is very difficult because the hands can't even get near each other. Plus, when used on the legs, it gives great access to "a cute" angle opposite the spreader.

out of sight, in a bind

A blindfold's importance to bondage deserves a chapter unto itself, but both the theory and application of one is so simple that a couple of paragraphs will suffice. Blocking the sense of sight increases the vulnerability the bottom feels and enables entrance into that most D/sireable of places in the solar system, "subspace." It also gives the top a chance to relax a bit, maybe make an adjustment in her underwear, and to climb down off the imaginary pedestal for a breather. A blindfold can greatly increase the sensation, and anticipation of sensation, that spankings, floggings, and tactile play with feathers and rougher objects deliver. Any cloth can be used to blindfold, plus there are many styles of premade blindfolds (like the free ones given on airplanes). Victoria's Secret has one in satin and lace that is Kitty Carlisle proper, or you can go to fetish shops and pick one up in leather or rubber. Be sure to use clean equipment, as the eyes are very susceptible to infection.

Bondage hoods or helmets, at the far extreme, can also be used to blindfold. They either have no eyeholes or have attachable blinders or zippers sewn in over the eye cups. (Whatever you do, *make sure your sub can breathe!*) There are safety precautions with blindfolds, of course: don't tie them too tightly—once again, for circulation reasons—and be careful if you are leading a blindfolded subbie around because removing the sight also seems to remove balance. But even more, a blindfold is a powerful psychological tool that can have unpredictable, even frightening effects on some. Hey, it's dark in there, so once you get it on your sub, watch any jokes about last cigarettes.

plastic fantastic

Tie wraps may sound like a spicy enchilada from Bangkok, but they are a most efficient way to strap somebody up. Also known as cable ties, these self-latching plastic straps were used by engineer types to hold wire in place before law enforcement officers caught on that they make great light-weight handcuff substitutes. They can be obtained from the local Radio Shack or other electronics wholesaler or ware-house in a range of sizes and lengths, from gargantuan to lil-liputian. They come in designer colors, including a shiny black that will coordinate well with your patent leather.

The little ones work well for toe bondage, but *do not* use them as cock rings. The pain of digging into an engorged member with side cutters is unbelievable (I'm told), and the downside of tie wraps is that after one use, they must be cut off, which will not get you bonus points with the local recy-cling committee. A reusable tie wrap that has a release latch does exist, but these are not as good for bondage because the same latch that makes them reusable makes them escapable. **Be very careful not to get tie wraps too tight**, because they can definitely and easily impede circulation.

packing straps

Relatively new to the bondage scene are very nifty little devices called packing straps. They are all the rage on back-packs, fanny packs, and the like. Packing straps are fastened with a unique male/female plastic clip, which is still adjustable when fastened. The beauty of these is that they can be con-nected in series, so you can line up as many as you need to strap down your strapping linebacker. A hint: you may have to tie a quick overhand knot at each buckle to keep the adjusting strap from sliding out under the constant strain of wriggling.

Still, this is easier than learning all those other knots. Choices of color, including patterns, build on the basic black.

wrap it up, i'll take it

Another innocent-looking and really fun bondage item is the shrink-wrap roller, available for a few dollars at mailing centers and U-Haul-type rental locations. The applicator is basically an easy way to apply yards and yards of Saran Wrap-type plastic to your lover. This also comes in different colors, and provides what is probably the easiest, most enjoyable bondage experience one will ever have. Your submissive sausage in full-body condom will be a wonderful, wrapped-up work of art. Stronger submissives can break through, so tying the joints at key contact points for reinforcement is wise. If they are tied underneath, they will not need to be tightly tied, because the plastic wrap will keep the bonds in place. Also, wrapping works better if you start with a naked subject, but be sure to leave erogenous zones uncovered for easy access (and be sure to stay away from the face!). Judging by the typical amount of perspiration, this may also be a good weight-loss regimen.

You can use a roll (or several) of Saran Wrap, but of course this is not as cost-effective. You can also use the stretchy plastic as a soft and forgiving rope substitute by simply bunching it up and tying your normal knots. Use pink for girls and blue for boys.

strip tease

For comfort, convenience, and camouflage, sometimes the best ties are ones you make yourself. Cloth, or even "pleather," purchased from a fabric store, about two yards long and cut into four-inch widths and folded over, is perfect. These ties can even be hemmed to prevent unraveling. When knotted and pulled tight, however, these can be hard to untie, so remember your slipknots. Leather and imitation leather can be used to hold metal O-rings at various bondage points along the limb, like makeshift manacles.

Ribbon, in a multitude of widths and colors, is a very festive way to tie up a loved one, making a lovely wrapped package. Some insist on at least 250 thread count for strength—the higher the thread count, the finer the quality and softness of the ribbon. I have at least two widths at my disposal: 3/4" and 1/4". The wider lends itself to most bondage situations, although you may want to take special care to "slip" your knots, for unless you do, ribbon is best untied with a knife. O-rings tied in place with ribbons are an elegant substitute for the manacle material listed above. Thinner ribbon works well on fingers and toes and is great for weaving a bundle of joy around your male masochist's member.

clothes stake the man

In a pinch, any long, soft article of clothing can be used for tying purposes. Stockings, preferably ones that are already ruined, are decent for this, and it will give your man a charge to be bound in something that earlier caressed your legs. Conversely, I love men in neckties, because I like where the neckties point, and I adore having a perfectly acceptable, built-in leash already on him. But the necktie can also be used as a tying strap. Most are long enough that you can tie a wrist and still have enough left to fasten to a bedpost in a spread-eagle tie, but if you come up short, just remember your sheet bend from chapter 4 to join two ties together. Be forewarned that heavy use in bondage can pretty much ruin a tie, so don't expect to use his Armani. But you can buy old neckties by the gross at yard sales (although the patterns are also pretty gross). Belts, too, can be used, but it seems the holes never line up with the buckles where you need them and a strapping male can sometimes break the cheap buckles they put on belts. Because of these failings, I prefer another kind of belt, a Black & Blue, accompanied with salt and a lime wedge.

crossing the line

As you progress in your skills, you may feel the need to have elaborate toys such as pillories and racks. Some get pretty complicated and they are always hard to explain ("Oh, our cotillion had a Spanish Inquisition theme this year!"). But an accessory like the X-shaped St. Andrew's cross, complete with eye-bolt tie points, can be a wonderful addition to your romping, especially once you get into the finer points of flogging. Each leg of the X gets a limb lashed to it, with the submissive facing either toward or away from the cross. Pay special attention to where X marks the spot. With the addition of wing nuts (and I am not just talking about you and your boyfriend) this device can be disassembled and stowed out of site, or used to hang bicycles in the garage.

nicolas caged

Bondage, taken to its most ridiculous extreme, can include full-coverage bondage accessories such as cages. Cages are a nonbinding way to imprison your lover. They can be purchased from bondage stores or catalogs, or you can use the larger folding metal dog kennels. However, because of the lack of tactile interaction with my slave, this *entre vous* method, for my tastes, really takes the *bon* out of bondage.

binding contracts

All of these bondage methods can be fun, and collecting the paraphernalia is part and parcel of the D/s experience. Although you may know more knots than a boatswain's mate, you will learn to appreciate the time you saved by not tying knots all the time. And, will you really feel you have that slave under your thumb until you clasp *his* in thumbcuffs and buckle that dog collar around his neck?

d/tails:
all trussed up
with no place to go—
a story of o-rings

Here is an example of how you can incorporate the other ties described in this chapter with rope to create an elegant yet economical, very versatile bondage ensemble.

You will need:

- **EIGHT** yards of 250-thread-count, two-inch-wide satin ribbon cut into one-yard lengths. Color is optional, but black is always in good taste. If your budget permits, two-inch-wide strips of kid leather are an excellent substitute.

- **ELEVEN** 1 1/2-inch chrome O-rings (any hardware store has these).

- **SIX** double-ended, spring-loaded chrome clasps (also in hardware stores, next to the O-rings).

- **THREE** 1 1/2-inch split-rings (like heavy-duty key rings, also in the same department of hardware stores).

- **ONE** three-foot pole ("spreader bar"). It can be a one-inch wooden dowel, metal tubing, or even one-inch PVC pipe. Drill three holes big enough to accommodate the split rings near each end, and one in the center, and sand any rough edges.

- At least **ONE** ten-foot length of 1/4- or 3/8-inch rope, with ends whipped.

- **ONE** sub, suitably dressed (or undressed) to your satisfaction.

- **ONE** roll duct, gaffer's, or adhesive tape; optional.

Before you start with your subbie, fit the split rings through the holes drilled near the end and center of your spreader bar. Be careful not to break a nail trying to negotiate the split rings.

Show a little affection to your sub, and then begin by taking one of the chromed O-rings and one yard of ribbon. Loop the ribbon through the O-ring and around the upper arm of the sub, just above the elbow, at least twice (or as many times as the circumference of the arm will allow). Make it tight, but still loose enough to be able to slide the ring under the ribbon and leave enough ribbon to finish in a slipped square knot, or a full bow knot if you are feeling festive. Repeat this on the other arm, and at each wrist, each ankle, and just above each knee. When finished, your sub will have eight ringed tie points on each limb near each of the major joints, which can be used in a variety of ways to restrain your sub.

Have your sub kneel. Fasten two of the double-ended clasps together and use them to join the O-rings on the bonds above the elbows behind the sub's back. If the anatomy allows, one clasp can be substituted. One clasp is used to fasten the wrists, also behind the back. Before clasping the wrists, slide the clasp through another O-ring. This will become of use later as a tie point. Spread the legs of your kneeling sub and hook each ankle to the split rings at the end of the spreader bar using the double-ended spring clasps.

Next, take a length of rope and the two remaining O-rings and make a crotch tie on your sub. Thread an

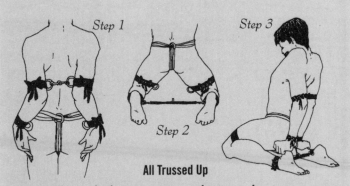

Step 1

Step 3

Step 2

All Trussed Up

O-ring through the rope so it ends up in the exact center. Placing that O-ring just below the navel of the sub, take the two running ends in opposite directions around his waist to the small of his back. Thread the two running ends through the remaining O-ring and continue on around the waist to the front ring. Thread both running ends (still in going opposite directions) through the O-ring on the front, then go between the legs and on either side of the genitals, up between the buttocks, and through the O-ring at the small of the back. Go back through the legs, retracing the same path, and tie off to the front O-ring with either a slipped square knot, or, if there is enough leftover rope, two adjustable taut-line hitches (one in each running end). This should be quite tight.

Take one of the remaining spring clasps and clasp the O-ring on the wrist clasp to the split ring in the center of the spreader bar, ending up in a position similar to the "camel pose" (see chapter 11). If you want, you can tape the spring release of the clasps for added security, as a dexterous sub can release them. You can finish with tape over the lips, if you choose.

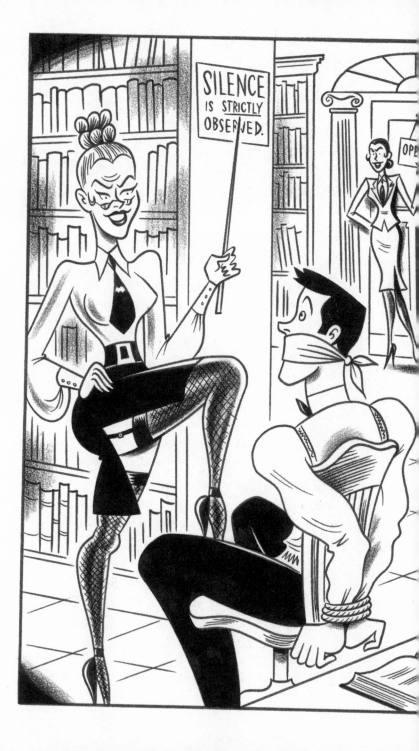

- 6 -

SILENCING
YOUR LAMB

gag rules

If bondage can be thought of as a hug by proxy, then its correlative surely is the gag as a kiss. Few bondage devices are as powerful or as dangerous, so very, very special caution must be given. I almost always gag my slaves though, even if I have a sub who is sworn to silence, or a screamer in a place where his cries have no chance of being heard. A gag is the exclamation point on bondage indignation, and as a rule, nothing so extends your affected domination of a favored pet as the ability to remove the expression of vocal communication.

On a less lofty level, gags are a hoot, from the movie *The Russians Are Coming* to the pilot episode of *That Girl* to the Antonio Banderas launcher, *Tie Me Up, Tie Me Down*. An alternate meaning of gag is "joke" (literally "routine" in Yiddish), and as such, comic appeal can be considered one more weapon in the arsenal of the top. All kidding aside, I am quite sure that if your sub is not asthmatic, he will have a more pleasurable bondage experience if comfortably gagged. And, just like biting a bullet, it will help him endure more of your delicious torture. It also prevents a SAM (Smart-Ass Masochist) from doing what is known as "topping from the bottom."

mouthing off

There are a number of very basic and very easy mouth mufflers available, both tangible and intangible. For example, a cocktail (or several), might be considered "chemical bondage." A cutting comment can be used to quiet. Sometimes, even a simple raised eyebrow from a powerful dominatrix such as myself can be more silencing than a stuffed handkerchief. I have witnessed some otherwise smarmy submissives intellectually bound and gagged trying to have a coherent conversation with, say, the polysyllabic William F. Buckley, Jr. But the gags I'm talking about are actual stuffings in the mouth, so think of this as a discussion to end discussion, but definitely not failure to communicate.

shut up, already

In movies and the golden era of television, the slightest slip of sheer fabric tied over or between some captive's lips is enough to stifle all sound, even if a potential rescuer is only on the other side of a curtain. A small piece of tape, lightly applied to the lips, seems to stop all sound and miraculously cannot be pushed out with the tongue. Unless your gullibility level is such that you don't think that professional wrestling has choreographed outcomes, you know full well that this isn't physically possible. This is not to say that the above-mentioned lightweight gags don't have their place. As a dominatrix, it is not necessary for me to always completely quiet my subs, just to let them know that one more aspect of their lives is being controlled by *moi*. If I am tying up someone in an artistic fashion, sometimes that crisp white dinner linen pulled between the lips and tied with a perfect square knot behind the neck is just the look I want, whether or not it lets some sound escape.

having a ball

One of the safer gags, believe it or not, is the classic ball gag, currently making a return to popularity due to the resurgence and retro appeal of fifties pinup queen Betty Page and the recent landmark film *Pulp Fiction*. As Bruce Willis detractors can attest, there is a certain comic appeal to seeing the lips of your sub spread and the mouth filled with a colored rubber ball. Technically, though, the beauty of the ball is the (near) impossibility of swallowing the gag, which can be fatal, and this is no joking matter. Choking, yes; joking, no. You can pick these up in fetish stores and sometimes even adult bookstores, usually on the shelf beside the dildos. But you can also make them yourself, which is much more economical than buying them. You can put the money you save toward buying a pair of Manolos, which you can't make yourself.

Any mouth-size rubber ball that is too big to swallow will do, although very hard rubber balls and the "superball" variety are not good ideas because of the tendency of the rubber to chip in small, dangerous pieces. The softer ones are also easier on teeth and dental work. The ball should be big enough just to fit behind the front teeth of your silent partner, although it is advisable to have a variety of sizes. A smaller one should certainly be used if your partner has any problem with the temporomandibular joint (where the jaws, neck, and ear meet). A strap with a buckle, a nylon luggage strap, or even a piece of ribbon can be threaded through a hole drilled through the very center of the ball. Drilling lessens the chances of splitting the ball, but if you are careful you can make a slit for your strap with a small knife or letter opener. Since the ball gag is reusable, it is necessary to practice good hygiene. Watch where you set it down when it is not in use. Because the ball is porous (and has a strap hole), washing it with soap can leave a bad-tasting residue, so when cleaning up, rinse with water only. You can semisterilize the ball by soaking it in vodka after each use. Call brands are not necessary, well brands will do.

If you decide to go the professional route and purchase a ball gag, you can advance to what is known as a *trainer,* literally a harness for the head that holds the ball gag in place, while supplying other straps to hold the jaw in place and offering O- and D-rings for attaching other bondage devices. Trainers often have blindfolds or blinders built into them as well. Ball gags come in a variety of colors, and for the very fashion conscious can become one more fashion statement. One particularly poignant memory I have is of my Bucks County friend Henry tenderly sliding a Tiffany-blue ball gag past his wife's Chanel-rouged lips, bringing out the azure highlights in her eyes.

getting serious

Besides the round rubber ball gag, other shapes can be used to fill the mouth. Bit gags, made out of leather or even metal, fit perpendicularly to the mouth and are a good choice if your slave cannot stand having large objects pushed past his teeth. As can be guessed from their very equestrian look, bit gags are the kind of accessories used in "pony training," an advanced role-play scene where slaves very literally horse around. A shape that is very popular, for obvious reasons, is the dildo gag. These come in a variety of lengths, but the longer ones are tough to, ahem, swallow. Go with the short, thick version for the mouth and leave the longer ones for other choice openings. Dildo gags also come double-sided. That is, one side is a dildo for the mouth and the opposite side is a dildo that protrudes from the other side of the mouth covering. Imagine the delightful possibilities of your tied and gagged lover trying doggedly to put that protrusion to work.

Other gags include the ring variety, which hold the mouth open by way of a large padded metal ring that is strapped into place. The benefit of this padded ring is that it still allows you access into the mouth of the slave while allowing the slave more access to air than other gags do. However, since air and objects can easily go in, saliva can more easily come out of rings, so be careful of the drool factor.

Leakage is much less of a problem with inflatable pump gags. Probably the most effective gag, a rubber bladder is put into the mouth and pumped up to fill the void using a hand pump not unlike the one on a blood-pressure monitor. These are often incorporated into bondage helmets that cover the entire head.

Another very effective gag is one in the actual shape of the inside of the mouth (more or less like a thick half moon). If you really get into this, you can take modeling clay, Play-Doh, or, in an effort to use something that doesn't taste quite so bad, several pieces of sugarless bubble gum, and get an impression of the inside of your sub's mouth, much like the procedure for dental bleaching trays and athletic mouthpieces. (In fact, two athletic mouthpieces, one for the upper teeth and one for the lower, glued together, make a decent form-fitting mouth filler). Once you get the basic shape from this model, you can go whole hog (or whole cow) and get a personalized gag made out of leather at a custom fetish store. But I digress from the practical to the sublime.

don't eschew fetish

You can incorporate your sub's (and your own) various fetishes into your gagging routine. Fetishes are deeply rooted in the mind and sexual psyche, so when a fetish item is thrust in the mouth, the taste and smell can overwhelm the slave with pleasure. Panty lovers like nothing better that the underwear of their domme stuffed in their mouth (either freshly laundered or freshly worn). Foot fetishists may love to have Mistress's stocking stuffed in his mouth, or even a ladies' tennis sock, again fresh from the laundry basket or from the foot. There are even strappy trainers, specifically designed to force the toe of a high-heeled pump into the mouth as a gag and hold the aromatic inside of the shoe vamp over the face and nose of the slave. And although the majority of fetishists seem to be male in gender, the ladies are not without their loves. I have seen many women go just gaga over having designer scarves tied on their limbs and in their mouths. There is no denying that a knotted Hermès silk print cravat holding a rolled and very sheer Wolfold stocking between the pouty lips of a beautiful subbette is *très chic*. However, since lipstick stains are very hard to remove from expensive fabrics, this may be a time for your silenced and stylish pet to go bare-lipped. You may want to add a dab of your perfume to the scarf as your scented signature.

let's listen to the tapes

Additional choices for silencing your submissive are adhesive tape, duct tape, or for those who want the best, motion-picture-gaffer's tape. Gaffer's tape is made out of a cloth with a tighter weave and a less permeable glue than duct tape. Duct tape's advantages are its incredible stickiness and its relative low cost. When tape is used, it is not necessary to actually have anything in the mouth, which can be helpful if your bottom has a overactive gag reflex. Once again it must be stated that just tape will not completely silence your lover, but it will impede speech and remind him just who is in charge. You can, however, use multiple layers of tape, at slightly different angles, to increase the efficacy of the gag.

When using tape to cover the mouth, a nifty trick that helps you remove it quickly is to fold over the last quarter inch on one side. This gives a little handle with which to pull off the gag when it is time to put your slave's mouth to other uses. As part of your dominating style, you can decide if the tape should be pulled off fast and painfully, like ripping off a Band-Aid, or slowly and painfully. The face skin is sensitive, so do try to be humane, occasionally. A good idea for cleanup is to keep a bottle of light oil (like baby oil) in your domme box. It will help remove any tape residue from the lips and face of your pet.

The most famous tape gag in BDSM history, and a cute thing to try on your sub, is the hidden-gag trick from John Willie's graphic novelette *The Missing Princess*. In the book, a very sheer handkerchief is tied between the lips and around the head of sub Sweet Gwen, and white adhesive tape is smoothed over the top of this. A flesh tone is achieved by applying makeup over the tape, and then lips are actually drawn on with lipstick. I once substituted wax lips for the lipstick and the 3-D effect was astonishing. This is an easy feat to duplicate at home, and with a veil to further camouflage the muzzle, you can take your silenced partner out in public for a movie (although sharing the popcorn will be tough for them). In cold weather, hands cuffed under an old-fashioned muff complete the bondage ensemble.

candy is dandy

Another tasteful way to plug the mouth of your playmate is my own creation, the candy gag. Candy gags, literally what the name implies, are not only in good taste, but taste good. An added advantage to candy gags is your submissive's breath will be much sweeter for the after-bondage kiss.

Hard candy, such as jawbreakers or Cherry Tissot, wrapped in a stocking works better than Godiva chocolates or other soft, melting confections. The stocking, or a piece of cheesecloth if one must make do, is necessary to hold multiple pieces of these small candies in place, thus preventing them from doing the trachea tango. I also recommend Callard and Bowser's Altoids (which is also the only candy that already has a dominatrix in the ad campaign). The peppermint, and especially the wintergreen, are good choices if you are feeling cruel. If you are feeling punitive, keep them in their metal box.

the last word on gags

Tasty mouth-fillers cause the production of saliva, which can start the choking process, so please *proceed with caution* when using them. Other, more traditional gags, such as wads of cloth, or even the finest Ritratti panties, while each having their own unique charm, can also have a way of working down the throat, so be careful and always be aware of your sub when you have a gag in their mouth. Never, repeat, *never* leave a sub when gagged, and don't have them gagged for extended periods of time. Always have a safe word, or, more likely, since they will not be able to talk, a safe sound (like humming "Figaro" or the opening strains to Beethoven's Fifth). This gives the bottom a way to bail out if he or she is choking or just having too much of a good time. But don't let these most basic safety precautions deter you from making your submissive a living embodiment of the statement, "A slave should be seen and not heard."

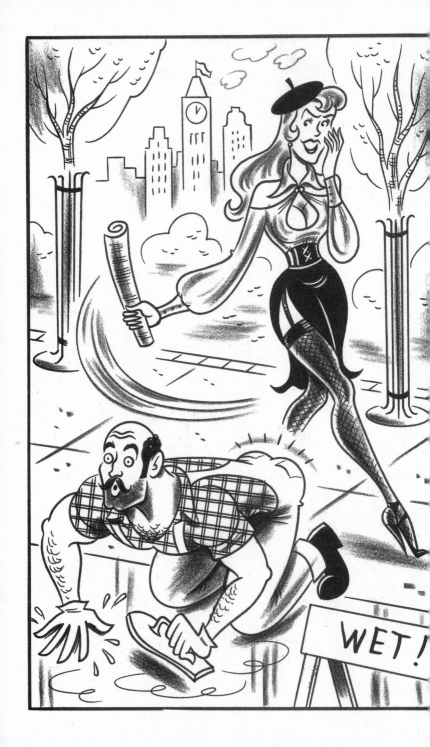

- 7 -

SPARE THE ROD, SPOIL THE MOOD

crack that whip

Let the bitch be your love, St. Bridget your saint,
Never flinch from a rod, or think of a faint,
Swish—swish—let it fall, till the glow of desire
Will run thro' your senses, and set them on fire.
                              —THE PEARL, EXCERPT FROM
                                "THE SPELL OF THE ROD"

Whip. The sound of the word is even whiplike, commencing
with the languid *wh* and ending with the staccato *p* sound. Be
it crop or flogger, switch or paddle, the instruments for corporal administrations are as rich and varied as the opportunities for their use. For the purposes of this chapter, the term
whip is loosely used to describe a wide variety of devices used
for corporal stimulation.

The *act* of whipping is considered depraved by most—a person unleashing his most primal aggressions on a helpless and
undeserving victim—and I do not wish to give the impression
of condoning such barbaric behavior. But you should be aware
that the use of whipping as an element of lovemaking was
known even to the authors of the *Kama Sutra* as a good thing
to incorporate in the bedroom. However, before we get into toys
and implements, let's look at the root of all whipping, the
spank. For spanking is to the whip as bondage is to manacles.

More people than you might imagine enjoy a little spanking in the privacy of their bedrooms, although they don't have
the slightest interest in the stereotypical "whips and chains"
image of BDSM. For the rest of you, a person's posterior is
one of the most looked at yet most frequently overlooked

erogenous zones. One of my greatest pleasures is demonstrating how a good spanking wakes up neglected nerve endings, enhancing the derriere's sensitivity and responsiveness. A properly executed spanking can bring your partner as much pleasure as your ministrations to more traditional areas.

spank you, spank you very much

One of the easiest ways to introduce BDSM to your partner is by adding a little slap and tickle to your foreplay. Easy, fun, free, and safe, what could be a more perfect activity? Everyone has a hand and everyone has a backside, therefore, no purchase is required.

If you are already incorporating a little role play into your lovemaking, spanking is a logical next step. If there is a more appropriate punishment for a bad Catholic schoolgirl or a less-than-fastidious maid, I can't think of it. Spanking can also be easily introduced as punishment for minor transgressions like leaving the toilet seat up or wearing white after Labor Day. Whatever your motivation, a well-done "over the knee" (abbreviated OTK in the personals) can turn any can into a can-do.

bun warming

Set the tone for the experience ahead by carefully choosing how you will expose your submissive. A brusque "Strip, you lazy slut boy," sends a very different message than if you dim the lights and slowly pull his pants down, massage his behind, and give it an occasional love tap.

Once your submissive is mentally prepared, your next task is to position him in a manner that makes him both accessible and aesthetic, derriere facing out, of course. How you do this is solely a matter of *your* preference, unless he has health concerns that must be addressed. You can drape him over your knee, on his hands and knees, or simply lying face-down on a bed.

As you begin, warm up your hand and his bottom with a series of light strokes on the entire buttocks. Reduce the stress on your hand by cupping it slightly; using a flat hand can hurt you as much as it hurts him. If you have delicate hands like I do, leather gloves will help prevent bruising—just one more reason why they make the perfect fashion accessory.

After a few minutes of hand-to-cheek contact, stop and treat your submissive to some light caresses. By now, his buttocks will have a lovely rosy glow, and you should take some time to admire your handiwork. Let your fingers occasionally drift between his legs to let him know this is hurting you more than him. Once he is assured you are not going to get medieval on his ass, you can begin to vary your routine by concentrating on specific areas and by increasing the intensity of your strikes, remembering to pay careful attention to how he responds and for signs of discomfort.

true confessions

No institution has played as important a role in perpetuating the day-to-day cycle of guilt, punishment, repentance, and a quick swat on the butt as the Catholic church (which is probably why most dungeons are empty on Sundays). For many people, their first introduction to this cycle is in parochial school. In the course of researching this book, I interviewed my former religion instructor, Sister Mary Michael.

PP: What is the purpose of spanking in Catholic education?

SISTER MARY MICHAEL: The purpose of spanking in Catholic education is to insure a prompt and painful reprimand for all transgressions committed by schoolchildren.

PP: When is the proper time to reprimand a transgressive schoolchild?

SISTER MARY MICHAEL: The proper time to reprimand a transgressive schoolchild is immediately after a transgression is detected or suspected.

PP: Where is the best place to spank a transgressive schoolchild?

SISTER MARY MICHAEL: The best place to spank a transgressive schoolchild is on the buttocks, midway between the upper thigh and the hip.

PP: What formation should the hand have when spanking a transgressive schoolchild?

SISTER MARY MICHAEL: The hand should be cupped for punishing minor transgressions of schoolchildren. The hand should be flat for punishing major transgressions of schoolchildren.

PP: Are there any acceptable substitutes for the hand?

SISTER MARY MICHAEL: Under Vatican II, both the ruler and the pointer were deemed acceptable substitutes for the hand. Both of these are more stringent instruments, and have the added benefit of being applicable to the knuckles, which Pope Paul VI deemed an acceptable substitution for the buttocks.

PP: What is recommended when a transgressive schoolchild appears to enjoy his prompt and painful reprimand?

SISTER MARY MICHAEL: If a transgressive schoolchild appears to enjoy his prompt and painful reprimand, the rite of exorcism should begin immediately. He is certainly the spawn of Satan, and otherwise, his soul is doomed to a lifetime of reckless abandon and an eternity of damnation.

whip it, whip it good

Whips are tools for an elaborate form of sensory play. Most submissives allow themselves to be whipped because they crave sensation. A properly ministered whipping invigorates the muscles and is good for the circulation in the same way as shiatsu massage. In addition, the touch of your lightest caresses will be intensified, and his skin will achieve the same rosy glow as after a good seaweed-and-oatmeal body slough. On a psychological level, whipping provides a catharsis for the bottom because the intense physical stimulation helps to subdue conscious thought—the perfect thing for Type A personalities. Whipping is almost always done in conjunction with its first cousin, bondage, for even the most willing of participants tends to stray if not anchored properly—and obviously, the target remaining stationary is of utmost importance.

pain puppies and pavlov

I don't mean to suggest there aren't people who wish to be whipped in order to experience pain. While you are certain to run into types like this, particularly at polka festivals and the first half hour of any neighborhood yard sale, this is an area for advanced study and not for us to address here. For now, consider corporal administrations a means solely to stimulate rather than hurt.

While many submissives (and a handful of dominants) are content with spanking as the apex of their BDSM activities, some enjoy the endorphin rush that can arise from engaging in more vigorous activities. Endorphins are neurotransmitters, natural narcotics your body releases to combat pain. High levels of endorphins create a euphoric feeling, described in the athletic world as a "runner's high." These same endorphins that are released by strenuous exercise are also released when you are put in pain, to enable you to adapt to physical impact and trauma. After the first time someone deliberately experiences pain, it is as if the body "understands" those impacts are not truly injurious so it doesn't have to protect itself. The same is true with the pain. The body apparently learns to send out endorphins immediately to reduce painful sensations. It is important to note that people who are enjoying an endorphin rush will need special attention as it begins to subside. Be prepared with a warm blanket and loving words to help bring your partner back to reality.

d/tails:
mistress payne's whine chart

Choosing the right instrument for an occasion takes the same skill and expertise as selecting the right wine to go with dinner. The dazzling array of varietal differences, as well as considerations such as the type of sound it makes, or the marks it leaves, can overwhelm the novice dominant, so use this chart when considering a new whine for your cellar.

TYPE	Equestrian Whips
KIND	Training whip, riding crop, stinger, quirt, popping crop, biting crop, dressage whip, dogging bat, jump bat
MATERIALS	Cowhide
CARE	Clean with a combination of saddle soap and a little water. Never oil your whips, as it will soften the leather. Relatively rigid, short to midlength whips like these are easily stored in pool-cue cases, architect tubes, or PVC piping.
MARKS	Crops: Wide, deep bruises Stingers: Tiny, red blotches
SOUND	Whoosh
SUMMARY	Crisp, lively, and classic. These whips make a statement with their presence alone.

TYPE	Multitailed Whips
KIND	Floggers, cat-o'-nine-tails, British navy cat
MATERIALS	Horsehair, rubber, plastics, rope, woven fabrics, metal chain, bolo cord, bison, bull, moose, lamb, deerskin, garment leather
CARE	Best left hanging, so be sure your items have a looped handle. Carefully wash your floggers with saddle soap, using cold or lukewarm water, and let dry. Generously spray with 70 percent isopropyl alcohol and again, let dry. Condition with Neet's Foot oil according to manufacturer's suggestions.
MARKS	When lightly applied, makes a lovely, light flush on the skin. More vigorous application can result in noticeable red lines that mimic the width and shape of the strands.
SOUND	*Thud*
SUMMARY	Big and focused; capable of creating a wide range of sensation. A properly balanced flogger should be a staple in your D/s toy chest.
TYPE	Single-Tail Whips
KIND	Bullwhip, stock whip, yard whip, black snake, signal whip
MATERIALS	Shaft: Nylon, kangaroo hide, horsehide, cowhide, red ride (tanned cowhide that is heavily oiled during processing, turning it red)

	Cracker: Waxed cotton, nylon twine, Kevlar, silk, male horsetail hair
CARE	See "Equestrian Whips" for cleaning. Store in a cool, dry place.
MARKS	Thin red stripes, welts, blisters
SOUND	*Keerack!* "Hey, that HURTS!"
SUMMARY	Concentrated sensation, often with an after-burn that kicks in on finish. Best when applied after a cowhide flogging.
TYPE	Not Whips at All
KIND	Paddles, batons, canes, rods
MATERIALS	Paddles: cowhide, wood Batons, canes, and rods: rattan, plastic, nylon, polyethylene, birch, Delrin, bamboo
CARE	Natural, polished canes need an applied finish such as a linseed-oil-based varnish.
MARKS	Polished canes leave double tracks with a bruise between them.
SOUND	*Swoosh*
SUMMARY	Intensely sharp and focused. Complex, deep sensations, with a crisp finish.

crop till you drop

Crops are a D/sential. They are easy to use, easy to travel with, and relatively inexpensive. And they add just a touch of discrete malevolence to your personal aura.

Look for a crop that is wrapped in leather, or coated with rubber to protect the wire binding from contacting and damaging the skin. Its shaft should be made out of fiberglass rods or graphite, which will make it resilient (not too easy or too stiff to bend.) A crop's end tip comes in many different sizes and shapes to induce a variety of sensations. Make sure the tip is stiff and not floppy.

Crops require little special care, other than the same cleaning and sanitizing procedures you use on your other leather playthings. Occasionally, the tip may get bent. If this happens, you can flatten it again by pressing it under a stack of books, or, if you are in a hurry and the damage is not too extensive, place the tip under a towel and press a cool iron over it.

flog wild

Just as different tools cause different sensations, a difference in materials will have a significant effect on how a toy feels, so a sense of refinement should be developed if one is to chose the right tool for the occasion. Leather will gather more momentum than rubber or plastic, resulting in a sensation that feels more like a pound than a slap. This feeling is commonly referred to as "thud." Synthetic materials, like rubber and plastic, create the feel of surface sting on the skin.

In ascending order from mild to severe, the most common leather floggers are:

- **THIN PIGSKIN,** a very soft leather that elicits a delicious sound with virtually no pain, no matter how hard you strike with it. Recommended for novices and as a warm-up toy when you are ready to advance to more strenuous activities.
- **DEERSKIN AND ELK** are also soft, sensual leathers. Floggers made from these materials, except perhaps when they are used at full force, will produce the sensation of being buffed like the black paint on a vintage Rolls Royce.
- **HEAVY PIGSKIN** and soft calf leather have mostly thud and some sting.
- **NUBUCK,** a heavy cowhide leather with a slight nap on the finish that gives it a satiny appearance, produces considerable thud and a solid sting.
- **UTILITY COWHIDE**, bullhide, and, at the far extreme, thick latigo provide more impact than is appropriate for a novice, and also increase the likelihood of damaging your sub's skin. You should hold off on buying one of these for a while.

Whips and floggers can also be made from garment leather, kangaroo, buckskin, bull, and other materials such as nylon, rubber, plastic, cotton, rayon, and feathers.

flogistics

The length and width of a flogger's strands also affect the feel of a flogger. The length of the strands affects the throw of the whip by adding additional weight and changing its balance point, while their width affects the impact area and the force of the flogger. The shorter the strands of the flogger, the greater the velocity. So, if you are testing two floggers of the same material and strand width, the shorter one will produce more sting. Typically, floggers range from twelve to fifteen inches for close work through eighteen to twenty-two inches for medium range, although general-purpose floggers can be as long as thirty-six inches.

In general, the shorter the flogger, the easier it is to handle and the more accurate it is to strike. A flogger of eighteen to twenty-two inches is recommended for most general flogging, while longer floggers are very dramatic but typically not worth the extra effort. Generally speaking, the softer the leather, the shorter the whip should be. A whip of very soft pigskin at twenty-two inches would be difficult to swing and, worse, hardly felt. At twelve to fifteen inches, however, it would give a nice pleasant warming feel to your submissive and make a delicious sound.

Narrow strands produce a more intense feel than wider strands cut from the same material. This added sting occurs because each strand strikes at a greater impact per square inch than a wider strand.

When shopping for a new flogger, a hands-on approach is best. Hold the instrument by the grip and get a feel for its weight and character. Your weight, height, physical strength, and arm length will also help determine which flogger is best for you. Don't be misled by fancy designs, as it is the whip end that is important, not the pattern on the grip. The best of toys of this nature have counterweighted handles, which are easily discerned. Hold the grip between your thumb and forefinger, about midway on the grip, with the flogger's strands hanging. If the handle is counterweighted, it will perfectly balance on your finger.

Your first purchase should be a light, multistrand flogger such as pigskin or deerskin. Even if you get more experienced, it can remain in your collection as a warm-up flogger. Later on, you may want to add a medium-level flogger such as a garment leather or elk and one stinger, perhaps pigskin suede or a heavier leather than garment. A crop is nice for localized impact, and keeping a sub in line. In addition, the wand of the crop can serve as a mild cane to give some initial experiences.

"flogging, anyone?"

While all these considerations may appear daunting, there are many day-to-day activities that have transferable skills easily applicable to whipping your submissive to the heights of ecstacy. For example, a drummer can make an excellent caner if he is also kinky. Folks who play a racket sport—tennis, squash, racquetball—or golf or even baseball tend to have an instinctive feel for BDSM toys because they already how to swing a tool to make something happen.

The swing of a tennis racket is the same swing a crop requires. You don't want to slice the racket; that would miss the ball altogether. You must be aware of the angle at all times in order to place the ball where you want it. Like a racket, your crop should become an extension of your hand. Concentrate on how you move, stand, swing, and what it feels like when the tip connects. There is nothing like body memory telling you, "Yes! I hit the sweet spot!"

The best way to learn good flogging techniques is to have an experienced dominant demonstrate on *you* first. This is the BDSM corollary to the adage "Do unto others as you would have others do unto you." It's useful to note that many submissives and bottoms give as good as they get, and can be wonderful instructors as well. If you live in an area where there are active BDSM organizations and clubs, you have the option of adding to your skills by attending workshops or demonstrations on subjects of interest.

it don't mean a thing if it ain't got that swing

Control is the key to flogging. If your strikes can't be delivered accurately, you are simply flailing around, which will make you both dangerous and silly looking. The best way to practice is on a pillow or sofa bolster. A store mannequin or inflatable companion works well for this, too. Just use something other than a person to practice on when learning to handle a flogger. Practice. Practice. Practice.

While floggers can be exhilarating, they must be handled as carefully as you would a thoroughbred race horse. To this end, one of your main concerns is to keep the strands from tangling, as tangled strands will destroy your stroke. A sling-shot stroke works well if your flogger is not counterbalanced (and most commercial floggers are not). The slingshot is done by holding the grip in one hand and the strands in another, and stretching the strands taut just before you release and strike. Some people put their finger in the D-ring at the end of the grip (if there is one) or hold the flogger by its slip band (a band of leather attached at the end of the grip to be slipped over the wrist in case the flogger slips out of the hand). Both of these are bad practices and cause inaccurate strikes and little, if any, control over intensity.

If your flogger has a balanced handle, keep the strands neat by draping them over your shoulder, the grip in your palm so the flogger's weight is evenly distributed. When you swing, the motion will come primarily from the wrist, as in fly casting, and the natural weight and momentum of the strands provides the basic impact. If more force is desirable, the arm can come into play.

You can develop a nice steady rhythm by swinging the flogger from side to side in a forehand/backhand action, keeping the falls on an imaginary horizontal plane. This will help you create a consistent stroke. If your flogger is heavy, more force will be required to get it into motion. Your strokes should use a motion that combines the thrust of your wrist, forearm, and elbow; avoid using too much shoulder. Add a wrist snap after you feel comfortable with your rhythm. This will add a new sensation to the same flogger, and the falls will act more like a single tail instead of just brushing the flesh like an automatic car wash.

Strokes should be parallel or slightly transverse, rarely perpendicular. Perpendicular strokes invite "wraps," when the tips of the flogger extend past your designated target, wrapping around and striking elsewhere, like the soft organs below the rib cage, which are absolutely off limits. Learn how to barely touch the skin's surface with the tips of the flogger in a stroke, then work where a little more of the end of the strands strike, then a little more. The feel of the stroke changes with the amount of the strand employed, varying the amount of "thud."

Another stroke is the "towel" strike, a snapping action of the flogger (either overhand or underhand) as though it were a towel. This leads to a snapping action with the tips of the flogger striking on their endpoints. This is very sting-y and can add spice and variety to the strokes.

A "windmill" pattern can be used too, where the dominant stands to the side of the submissive and rotates the wrist quickly clockwise or counter clockwise to deliver very quick strikes. This is usually used on the buttocks. If you want to strike in patterns other than downward and have two matching floggers, a figure-eight pattern can be used. Deliver the strokes to the buttocks in a transverse pattern, first on one cheek and then the other. This technique can also be used on the back or chest.

Vertical throws work well if your submissive is facedown on a bed or bondage table. This swing will allow you to use gravity to impact more force, or simply let the falls drop softly from above, letting gravity do the work for you.

If your bottom is mounted high on a step-up St. Andrew's cross, the buttocks will be at an optimal position for horizontal strokes with a flogger. If your bottom is short, or on a floor-level cross, you will have to stoop down, or kneel to reach the sweet spot without altering your strokes dramatically.

A good dominatrix will start with a soft whip or light cropping for a warm-up before moving on to heavier floggers or toys. Slowly building up prepares your submissive and gives him time to adapt to this special attention. Warm-up is important even for the expert, since it gets the endorphins stirring, which makes the difference between erotic and nonerotic pain.

A good whipping is not like whisking eggs for an omelette, and one of the secrets for a successful execution is to always keep your submissive at the edge of anticipation by varying your routine. Be sure to stop occasionally and use the same soothing tones and gestures you've already employed when spanking. You can send your subbie on a pleasure ride by slowly dragging the strands of the flogger over his body; the neck works wonderfully as a handy erogenous zone for this. You can also play bad cop by doing this in reverse, with the last-minute substitution of a crop for a feather duster.

aural sex

The aural experience of being whipped can have a profound effect on a submissive, particularly if he is blindfolded. Each whip has its own sound, and it doesn't take long for someone to anticipate the impact of a lash by the noise it makes. Floggers, with their numerous strands, create sounds that are relatively soothing compared to that of a fine Australian bullwhip, whose loud crack is attributed to the popper breaking the sound barrier at a breathtaking seven hundred miles per hour.

single-minded

Single tails cover a wide range of whips from a small dog whip (the kind carried but rarely used by Australian shepherds) to the bullwhip, which should not be confused with the signal whip. The dog whip is usually short, three feet or less, and has a short tang on it. Typically, the tang (a piece of hard leather at the end of a single-tailed whip) should be replaced with something softer, as the original tangs can cut human skin unless used by an expert.

The quirt or horsewhip is made similarly to the dog whip but may be three or four feet long, while a signal whip (e.g., a dogsledder's whip) has a fine fabric fall (an extension of the whip tip) of six to eight inches. This whip is meant to crack and make a noise rather than strike. It is used in BDSM for striking, but should be used with great care because the fine fall can easily cut.

Other whips, like the border whip, black snake, and short bullwhips, can be very intense. The black snake is a lead-loaded whip meant to strike with a white-hot impact. A bullwhip is like the much smaller signal whip in that it has a long fabric fall. Like the signal whip, it was not made to strike directly but to crack and make a sound near the ear of a lead ox in a team. It is mainly used for effect in wrapping and cracking. Some expert individuals may use it to strike, but it is exceptionally dangerous to use and takes a wide space to swing. All but the most expert should stay away from bullwhips.

For most single-tails, kangaroo is the best leather since it is very resilient, but cowhide is used as well. The quality of the whip is indicated by the number and size of the strands woven to make it up. A whip woven with eight strands or plaits is typically very good. Some can be found with twelve and even sixteen strands, which is better. While whips with more strands have artistic value, the eight-strand is adequate for most uses.

Four, six, eight, twelve, fourteen, and sixteen plaits or braids are the most common configurations, although a craftsman can produce outstanding whips with up to twenty-eight plaits. While the plaits on single-tails are fine, the whip should *not* feel stiff as a board. Anyone can braid fine and tight, but a fine, tight braid that is also flexible when new is the mark of true craftsmanship.

With the single-tail, practice, practice, practice before you ever strike a human; its margin of error is much less than a flogger's. My criterion for demonstrating reasonable prowness is this test: Take five balloons and tie them to a string or a line across the room. You should be able to strike each of them and flip them around the string without breaking them and then strike all five and break each one. Once you have that much control and range, you are ready. Even then, have your submissive wear jeans or some thick garment if you are going to use a single-tail, as they can leave scars if improperly used. An intelligent submissive should always require to see the dominant use the single-tail before submitting to its use. If in doubt, decline.

pain, pain, go away

Flogging has many safety considerations. First and foremost: *never* strike someone out of anger. Never. Ever. Ever.

Never strike over any soft tissues; any dominant who says he can do it should be avoided. The buttocks, shoulders, and thighs are allowable, but the abdomen and the area between the bottom of the rib cage and the buttocks are dangerous, as kidney damage and worse can result. Avoid having the strands wrap around the submissive, since the added velocity often is too intense or can injure. Strike downward and not across the body.

Always have a safe word and be sure the dominant is ethical. It is best always to have a spotter, someone who can watch the proceedings and has the power to stop them if things look like they are getting out of hand. This should be a neutral party or someone the submissive knows and trusts. Use common sense and remember this is a *person* being struck.

Along with graver dangers, cuts and bruises can occur as the result of a vigorous session. Any broken skin should be immediately treated with 70 percent rubbing alcohol, applied with a sterile swab. Bruises can be ameliorated by using arnica ointment, available at most health-food stores. Never use arnica on broken skin.

Some would say that whipping is too dangerous and expensive an activity for a novice interested in sado-masochism. But I believe the benefits of a good whipping far outweigh any of its detractions. With high-quality instruments, ample practice, and a willing partner, you will be able to whip your love life into new heights of desire. Remember, there is always room for Flagell-O.

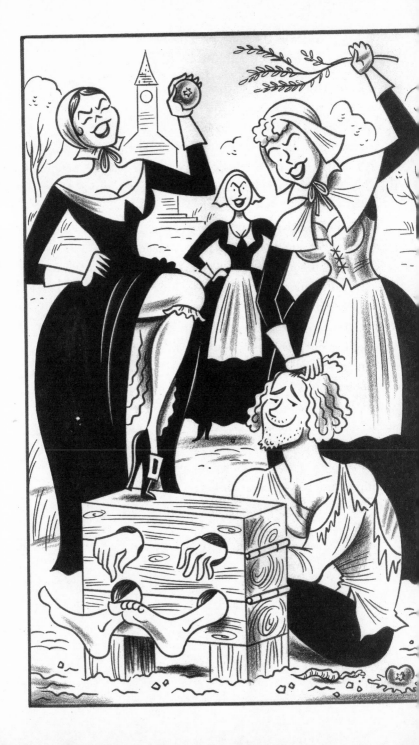

- 8 -

D/SENSE AND SENSIBILITY

dungeon decorum

It's Saturday night, you just invested your last paycheck on a pair of butter-smooth leather britches that make your backside look like Jennifer Lopez's. You don't want to waste that look in your basement. It is time to go out, child.

saturday night at the dungeon, who cares what spanking you see . . .

It ain't always what you do, but who you let see you do it.

—HOMER BANKS,
CARL HAMPTON, AND
RAYMOND JACKSON

Public BDSM clubs and parties can be great places to learn new skills, get ideas, or experiment with specialized equipment before investing in them for your home dun-geon. Submissives use these events as an opportunity to publicly demonstrate their devotion to their master or mistress, and they also provide tops with an opportunity to demonstrate their prowess in favored S & M techniques. Attendance at these venues also gives one another excuse to strut his or her finest fetish fashions.

The idea of going to one of these venues may seem daunting at first, particularly if you've ever had the misfortune of watching a stereotypical Hollywood BDSM scene.

On these sets, all the women are perfectly curvy and pervy, the men are dark and dangerous looking, and there is always a homicidal maniac on the loose, taking advantage of the sinister and seductive environment.

Fear not. Most people you encounter at a BDSM club or party are no more beautiful or exciting than people you meet anywhere else, so put away your fears of feeling like Linda Tripp at a Victoria's Secret catalogue shoot, and consider adding a bit of the dark side to your nightlife.

A dozen major cities from coast to coast have public BDSM clubs, and dozens more have BDSM organizations that host parties open to members and their guests. While East Coast gatherings tend to start and end later than their West Coast counterparts, here are some basic things to expect if your taste runs to this kind of adventure.

less libations, more abrasions

Once, a philosopher; twice, a pervert.
—VOLTAIRE

All body types are welcome, and I guarantee you will see more than one leather-clad person who looks ten times worse than you do on your worst fat day. However, standard operating procedure dictates that all bodies in attendance be twenty-one or older.

If you think you are going to be able to steel your nerves, or soothe your subbie, with a few stiff drinks once you get there, forget it. Most clubs have a premises-wide no-alcohol rule in effect. While this may appear to be overly cautious, do you want to be in the same room as a person with a stinger in one hand and their third *stinger* in the other? On the upside, this cuts down on your expenses for the evening, particularly when you consider women get free or reduced admission to many clubs.

the master of d/stiny

Not everyone at a club is there to participate. Plenty of people just come to dress up and socialize, while voyeurs and the simply curious are always well represented. But the most important people at any gathering are those in charge of safety, referred to as Dungeon Master/Mistress (DM).

These people are responsible for ensuring the equipment is in good working order, shared equitably, and that participants are safe at all times. DMs are willing to help instruct novices on the safe use of all equipment provided on the premises and also act as mediators if there are any scenes that have potential safety concerns. A DM is often the chief enforcer of the no-alcohol policy.

scene and be heard

Most public scenes last between a half hour and an hour. Doms who violate this unspoken rule run the risk of being perceived as vain or inept, and may, in either case, be quietly discouraged by the Dungeon Master. Dominants wishing to use popular items of equipment are also advised that reserving pieces with quarters or tokens, as one would a pool table, is frowned upon. For an acceptable substitute, savvy doms can queue their submissives while they pass the time in less tedious activities.

Good manners and quiet discussion are requisite behavior as the public scene unfolds. Chanting, "Hit 'im again! Harder! Harder!" is considered quite rude, as is leaving your beeper on, or choosing the wrong moment to call the au pair on your cell phone.

A general rule of thumb for all parties, whether public or private, is, "What's mine is mine and it remains that way unless I tell you otherwise." This rule applies to both equipment and submissives, with the one exception being toys and equipment provided by the host. In this instance, there is no need to be shy, although you must receive instruction on anything that is new to you. It is also acceptable to ask to borrow an attractive item, but under no circumstances should such permission be assumed. This rule also pertains to another domme's submissive, no matter how tempting the forbidden fruit.

It will probably surprise many of you reading this to learn that with the exception of the most Bacchanalian of private parties, sexual intercourse and other forms of penetration in public are not only frowned upon, but actively discouraged. People whose preferences run to more extreme forms of play also tend to be out of luck for most public activity, except on special occasions like giving a demonstration. If you enjoy messier activities such as playing with melted candle wax, you must take special measures to be a considerate guest and always get permission from the host before waxing poetic. Essential to staying in the hostess's favor is providing your own sheets of plastic in order to prevent nasty wax stains on the Kashan.

d/tails:
erector sets

As I mentioned earlier, one of the most compelling reasons to go to a club or party is the opportunity it affords to play with equipment you may not wish to have—or be able to afford—in your home. You are sure to encounter at least one St. Andrew's cross, a spanking bench, a bondage chair, and a number of other items at almost every venue you attend.

BONDAGE RACK: A large, horizontal wooden frame, about six feet high and four and a half feet across, that has a series of eyebolts along the sides. A bondage rack is perfect for intricate kinds of bondage, both constriction and extension, especially the complex crisscrossing of a spiderweb design. It can also be used as a substitute for a St. Andrew's cross or a regular rack for a flogging scene.

BONDAGE BED: A wooden frame, about seven feet long and three feet wide, with a latticed canvas bottom. This also has a series of eyebolts around the edge of the frame, which provide a myriad of options for a supine bind.

BONDAGE CHAIR: An oversized chair, usually wooden, but occasionally metal. These chairs often have built in wrist and ankle cuffs on the arms and legs, and have built-in openings or eyebolts so you can add additional ties. Some models have only very thin slots, but if you come prepared with black satin ribbon, you can be one of the few in the club able to make use of this lovely item.

ST. ANDREW'S CROSS: Unlike the traditional T-shaped Christian cross, a St. Andrew's cross is X-shaped, and handcuffs, rather than nails, are recommended. Many models have a step-up platform that raises your sub up to perfect striking height. The St. Andrew's cross is usually one of the most popular pieces of dungeon equipment.

RACK: Regular racks are shorter and stockier than bondage racks. They often do not come with eyebolts, although like the St. Andrew's cross, many have built-in restraints for both the feet and hands.

CATHERINE WHEEL: A solid wooden vertical wheel with restraint points that place your submissive in an X-position, and which also has a neck support for when it's time to revolve. When using this piece of equipment, remember you are a dominatrix, not a contestant on *Wheel of Fortune,* and care should be taken not to spin your subbie too vigorously.

SPANKING BENCH: Catholics will be reminded of kneelers, others of a massage chair. They are a comfortable way for you to safely and comfortably present your backside.

MEDICAL ROOM: Many clubs will have a separate area with a medical theme. These can range from an old OB-GYN table tucked in a corner to an elaborate setup that looks like a set from *ER*. Bring your own scrubs and speculum.

CAGE: There is something about a cage that appeals to a wide variety of people, from those into bondage to those into humiliation. Their wide range of sizes lend themselves to many different moods, from a low canine cage to a birdcage shape that is perfect for restraint a-go-go.

SLING: Canvas or leather slings are a great way to simultaneously suspend and expose your subbie. A well-designed sling will support your submissive's derriere and back, up to about the shoulders. See if it's adjustable so you don't strain yourself bending over to get to the interesting parts.

STOCKS: Heavy wooden stocks are popular among spanking and caning enthusiasts, as they ensure the immobility of the target. Unlike the stocks you recall from early American history, club stocks rarely have neck holds, although some come with a bench so both wrists and ankles can be restrained.

Now that you know the ups and downs of the bondage nightlife, finally, you have additional choices in answer to the eternal question, "Where in the world are we going to go this weekend?"

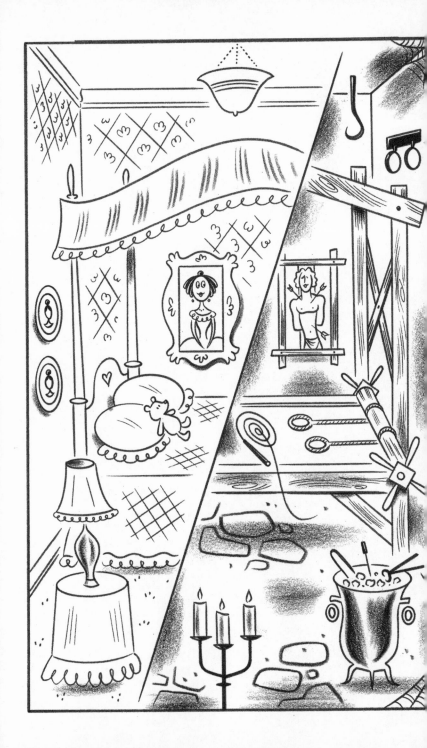

- 9 -

MASTERING THE BEDROOM

home atone

By your truth she shall be true,
Ever true, as wives of yore;
And her "Yes," once said to you,
Shall be Yes for evermore.

—ELIZABETH BARRETT
BROWNING, "THE LADY'S YES"

Whether you want to make him your love slave for an hour or the evening, you will find him more receptive—and the entire experience more pleasurable as a whole—if you take the time to create the right environment in your boudoir. Since most people cannot afford the cost or loss of living space to a room dedicated as a home dungeon, knowing how to have your bedroom serve a daytime function while at the same time being able to easily transform it into a nighttime pleasure dome is a skill you simply *must* acquire.

When you are on your home turf, you have the opportunity to carefully prepare and assemble everything you will require (unlike a date that ends up at a hotel or his place). Complete control of your environment is one of the keys to complete control over him.

D/s time is a time for privacy. Set your answering machine so it picks up on the first ring, and be sure the volume is turned all the way off. Cell phones and pagers, whether yours or his, should be tucked away until playtime is over. If you have a large, mean dog, this is a good time to tie him outside to keep your neighbor from wanting to borrow a cup of sugar at the wrong time.

cleanliness is next to dommeliness

Needless to say, your home dungeon must be tidy. He will be unblindfolded at some point, and there is nothing more likely to take him out of subspace then seeing the mishmash of clothing on the floor that was the result of your latest fashion crisis. Decide what you are going to wear ahead of time and put everything else away. If you plan on a change of clothing, put whatever you will require in another room so you can discreetly step out and slip into something less comfortable.

Put your Beanie Baby collection away for the time being. Same thing goes for anything else that is cutesy. You want to project the air of a dominatrix, not a giddy fifth-grader.

Wrought-iron accessories like candlesticks or lamps are relatively inexpensive, and can add a hint of severity to almost any bedroom. They also come in a huge array of styles, so you are certain to find a few items that complement your decor.

Candles are traditional and indispensable mood setters. Fire and safety considerations notwithstanding, you can never have too many candles. Invest in a few different shapes and sizes; stick with solid colors and sensual scents like cinnamon or sandalwood. Be sure to never leave lit candles unattended—and no, a bound and gagged slave will not do as an attendant.

striking a chord

Music can also have a profound effect on your environment, and there are a wide range of choices from classical to contemporary that can add a seductive and dramatic element to your domination. Here is a short list of some of my favorites.

MODERN MUSIC

Perfume Tree *A Lifetime Away* alternative pop-rock
Catherine Wheel *Ferment* industrial, alternative
Sisters of Mercy *A Slight Case of Overbombing* goth, rock
Andreas Vollenweider *Caverna Magica* New Age harp
Lords of Acid *Lust* club, techno acid
Dead Can Dance *Into the Labyrinth* gothic, club
Merzbow *Music for Bondage Performance*
     Japanese industrial
Coil *Love's Secret Domain* experimental, industrial
Mickey Hart *Planet Drum* ethnic fusion
O Yuki Congugate *Peyote* experimental, ambient
Enigma *Cross of Changes* Gregorian, club
Depeche Mode *Songs of Faith and Devotion* postpunk club
Cocteau Twins *Blue Bell Knoll* alternative pop
Nine Inch Nails *The Downward Spiral* club, industrial

SOUNDTRACKS

Passion, Peter Gabriel
Birdie, Peter Gabriel
Lost Highway, various artists (Trent Reznor, Angelo
     Badalamenti, Barry Adamson, Rammstein, etc.)

Star Wars Trilogy: The Original Soundtrack Anthology,
   The London Symphony Orchestra,
   John Williams, conducting
The Hunt for Red October, Basil Poledouris

CLASSICAL MUSIC

Orff *Carmina Burana*
Wagner "Ride of the Valkyries"
Holst *The Planets,* "Mars"
Bach *Toccata in D minor*
Verdi *Requiem,* "Dies Irae"
Mussorgsky *A Night On Bald Mountain*
Kitaro *The Light of the Spirit*
Chopin *Nocturnes*
Schubert *Piano Trio Opus 100,* second movement
Bach Cantata 50, *Nun ist das Heil und die Kraft*
Beethoven *Grosse Fuge*
Mozart *Requiem*
Chopin *Grand Polonaise*
Wagner *Tristan und Isolde,* "Liebestod"
Ravel *L'enfant et les Sontileges*
Saint-Saëns *Samson et Dalila,* "Baccanale"
Villa-Lobos *Bachiana Brasileras*
Stravinsky *The Rite of Spring*
Bartók *Duke Bluebeard's Castle*

a rope in time for thine

Plan and prepare for what you would like to do ahead of time. If tying him spread-eagled on the bed is in the future, attaching your handcuffs to the bed now will help you keep the flow of the evening seamlessly under your control. While you are doing this, you should also be considering what other toys or accessories you are going to want to use (or even think you may want to use), and assemble these all in one easily accessible place.

I believe that assembling bedroom equipment works on the same basic premise as setting a table—a place for everything and everything in its place. My equipment is always laid out like a place setting—blindfold, gag, wrist and or/ankle restraints, clamps, and any special toys I might require, like a dildo or a candle. And I always have two thick, fluffy towels and robes for later.

disguising your dungeon

Sometimes it is difficult to keep things accessible and at the same time well hidden. If you think BDSM may become a regular part of your love life, consider converting your bedroom into a dungeon that essentially works like a motion-picture set: easy to assemble and quick to break down when you're done.

For example, square tablecloths can be reversible, with the print of your choice for everyday use and a wonderfully solid black backing. Stitch a few velcro loops (fabric strips with velcro on both ends) along one side of the tablecloth, and you can quickly attach the loops around your curtain rod. This creates a dramatic background of black curtains, and it is easily kept out of sight when not in use for play. If the tablecloth reaches the floor, the space under the table itself can make an excellent storage place for rope and extra candles, which, by the way, keep the room smelling great.

If you are lucky enough to have a bedroom with a lidded window seat, with just a few eye hooks, the lid can be used to hang floggers or other items where tangling is an issue. Of course, there is ample storage for other items inside the seat.

Two well-placed hanging plants are great ways to disguise eyebolts in the ceiling that are convenient when you wish to flog but you don't want to take the time to assemble the St. Andrew's cross. They also work wonderfully for creating interesting extension or constriction bondage positions.

Having the proper pillow for each activity is also important. I would no sooner use a toss pillow to raise a well-shaped bottom than I would use a breakfast pillow after noon. Envelope pillows are great places to store small things, like gags or a small pair of clamps, and also are creative places to store condoms and K-Y jelly.

Of course, you do not need to confine your imagination and your interior-design skills to the bedroom. Different rooms in your home can lend themselves to a myriad of interesting situations and delightful dilemmas for your submissive.

While whips and chains are sure to get his attention, your thoughtful preparation for a few hours of pleasure is what will keep you remembered.

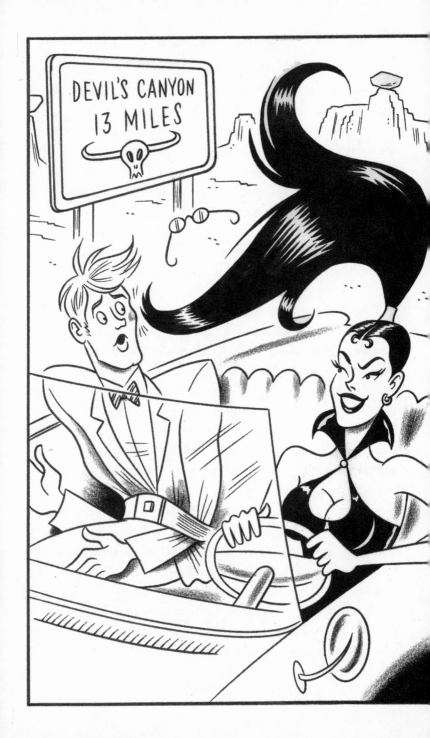

- 10 -

TAKING YOUR SHOW ON THE ROAD

location, location, location

Yet all experience is an arch, wherethrough gleams that
untravelled world, whose margin fades forever as I move.
—TENNYSON

Nothing aids adventure as much as a change of scenery.
Cinching down the safety belt and getting away with your
lover for your own production of *Abducted in Acapulco,*
Bound in Barcelona, Kidnapped in Katmandu, or just plain
Tied Up in Terre Haute is a wonderful way to add a little
umbrella to your sexual highball. But packing up your "trou-
bles" in your old domme bag can be trouble for you unless
you take certain precautions.

dante's baggage claim

I am quite certain that a special part of Hades awaits the
parties responsible for airplane hijackings. Perhaps nothing
has limited the range and mobility of the innocent fetishist
more than the security checks at airport terminals. The prob-
ing eye of the X ray scanner sees all and tells all to the under-
paid, overuniformed, undereducated security staff, who wait
to rifle through and drool over your very personal person-
ables, and always in front of your traveling companions
queued up in line to get to the gates.

Getting ready for these little friskings is good practice for
keeping one's dark side in the dark, not exposed to the harsh
light of some government agency's fluorescent lamps.
Traveling, especially traveling by air, can present problems, but

they are not insurmountable, and indeed, they can contribute to the excitement of the game of captivating lovemaking.

hide in plain sight

My motto on traveling with toys is simple: hide in plain sight. Some of my fetish stuff blends right in. But even more mundane travel gear has alternate uses. For instance, the shoulder strap of my Tumi carry-on bag, with its wide leather pad, makes a quite usable gag. There are all manner of quick-release packing straps (discussed in chapter 5) that can go on the outside of my bag, and these straps can bind arms and legs as well as luggage. My jump rope? Well, let's just say it can *keep* someone from jumping.

Separating some objects can make them look less suspicious. I keep my silk scarf collection in my underwear bag, where it is really hard to tell them from my panties. Plus, any male security officers checking my bag are likely to get uncomfortable when they start going through my drawers. My blindfold I keep in my soft side briefcase, and even when wearing it while sleeping in first class, it looks innocent enough. I take the strap out of my two traveling ball gags. If questioned, I show them how I use the balls for exercise equipment to strengthen my grip. These I pack with the jump rope, along with some wonderful wide, latex rubber bands that I also use in my workout and my slave's. The funny thing is, I do use all of this stuff to stay in shape.

saddle baggage

To travel hopefully is better than to arrive.
—Robert Louis Stevenson

Tina Wynn is a dear colleague of mine who is a traveling photographer and competing equestrienne. She has been on both sides of a bow tie and likes to keep up with a very diverse group of D/s friends and lovers. "When I travel for an equestrian event, the sky is the limit, of course. I mean, I have to travel with my gear . . . I can't just run out to Bits, Bonds, and Beyond to pick up new equipment in every town I visit. Pretty much no one ever questions crops, bridles, even cruel-looking gag bits and halters when I travel in this mode. And certainly my remuda of pony girls don't have a thing to say."

Handcuffs present a special problem, as they are considered a weapon that can be used to restrain victims during a hijacking. (And I vote for the flight attendant with the cute turned-up nose and the broad shoulders.) Traveling is a good time to substitute plastic tie wraps, which will not show up under the X ray. But, if you still insist on the metal kind, there are ways of getting them on. Tina once successfully got them aboard as a carry-on by using them to handcuff her attaché case to her wrist, as she professed the contents were industrial secrets and a security risk. Of course, the security officers had to go through the briefcase, but she had enough sealed film material in envelopes to make it look official enough. Still, checking is the better way to go with handcuffs. And don't think that will be completely safe, either. Several times my luggage has been tampered with while in the care of the airline baggage personnel. Once I even heard a noise in my bag and it turned out to be one of my vibrators that had been turned on. I know that luggage loader is still getting a laugh out of that one. I have since learned from that mistake, and pack the batteries in a separate plastic bag.

"My whips and crops travel in a tubular blueprint case," Tina continues, "which expands to fit my longest one. Even through the X ray scanner, nothing usually shows up, except for the metal studs in the handle of one of my crops. Sometimes I will put my floggers in individual dark stockings that go in the suitcase. Not only does it help camouflage the flogger, but it keeps the little strands of leather from entangling with each other."

Without a cover like Tina's, sometimes the best way is just to FedEx your kinky toys to your destination ahead of you, if your budget permits. This is especially true if you are crossing any national borders. And beware of Canada. Our friendly neighbor to the north will confiscate anything they consider pornographic, even scholarly literature on the subject, and you will be listed in their computers as a possible sex offender. Which, by the way, makes a splendidly kinky line on your electronic greeting cards.

letting the cat out of the bag

Some of my friends have not been as lucky when trying to get through security checks. Judy L., a building manager in Chicago, was once returning to O'Hare from Denver.

"As my bag was going through the X ray at DIA, the

security officer, after pondering the image on the television screen for a few moments too long, asked if he could inspect my bag. Of course, I was already running late (as anyone who flies through DIA always is) and I had no time to argue. The first thing he pulls out is a rather large double-ended dildo.

"'What's this?' he asked.

"'It's a dildo, you dildo,' I said, louder than I had to. 'And this is a riding crop, and this is a flogger, and this is a butt plug,' I announced as I threw sex toys left and right on the table. 'I don't think I could take a plane over with any of them, do you?'

"Well, his face turned pretty red, and he just said, 'No, ma'am,' and he left me to collect my belongings and move on. Everyone in line had a good laugh. But I'll tell you, I got no less than three offers for dinner in Chicago flying back on the plane."

Sometimes there is an advantage to letting secrets out.

Even if your road trip is by automobile, it pays to follow some of the above precautions. The weirdest stuff can happen: breakdowns, questionable searches by local law-enforcement officers, even innocent occurrences like your luggage ripping open and spilling the contents. A little bit of camouflage keeps the *bon* in *bon voyage*.

s & m-acgyver

Of course, sometimes you will find yourself in a traveling situation where you don't have your toys but you do have a boy toy (I am quite certain there is a Murphy's Law that covers this) and the need to improvise will arise. Believe it or not, you are surrounded by items that can very easily, with just a little practice, be turned into a cornucopia of D/s items.

I have already discussed with you the great cuffs used on exercise equipment and the use of clothing and belts as bondage material. Another very basic, very easy idea I have used from time to time is right under your tush, if you are seated on the hotel bed. Mental institutions and hospitals for years have prided themselves on their wet sheet ties as almost inescapable. So, taking a cue from them, you can take the bottom of your hotel sheet and rip it into two inch strips. You will have a very handy supply of strapping material that is—relative to, say, a phone cord—quite comfortable. Fitted sheets will not work for this, but hardly any hotels use fitted sheets. Be sure to leave the bed made when you finish, and pick up all the strings that will be left behind (or better yet, let subbie do it). No one will be the wiser, even the next person who is short-sheeted, as the inches you take off will hardly be noticed.

Need to silence your playmate? The crisp white linen from your room service will hold your rolled-up panties, or that gigantic chocolate-covered strawberry, securely in his mouth. Fold the napkin so any lipstick stains won't show when you leave it on the tray outside your door.

instant cool whip

You have found resourceful ways to restrain your pet, now what? You can make a economical, environmentally sound flogger from an ordinary bungee cord. Take off the hook (unless you are a true sadist) and peel back the fabric covering the bungee cord, exposing sort of a cat-o'-nine-tails of rubber dreadlocks. With tiny cuticle scissors, you can make short work of the sheathing, doubling it back halfway to form a handle.

If passion has taken over and you do not have time for the bungee trick, you can make a handy and quite effective quirt out of the cardboard tube used on a wire pants hanger. These work wonderfully, especially if you have very full, very arched eyebrows, broad padded shoulders, and open-toed platform shoes. And no one would ever suspect that such an innocent-looking tube of cardboard could be such an instrument of inquisition. Be very careful, for these can easily create contusions quicker than you can say "Mommie Dearest."

Another handy faux flogger is a dime-store bamboo back scratcher. I have used the flat back of that little hand to almost blister myself out of one relationship. It makes a wonderful slapping sound and, of course, is great for getting to that hard-to-reach itch between my shoulder blades when subbie is indisposed.

There are a lot of locker-room jokes made about towel popping, but a properly made rat-tail is a formidable weapon, *if* it is folded and rolled correctly. To do this, fold the two corners of one of the long sides over to the midway point of the opposite long side to make a wide triangle. (Your towel will

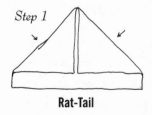

Step 1

Rat-Tail

look like the silhouette of a large gable-end house). Starting at the tip of the "roof," roll the towel tightly along either of the roof's ridges down to that ridge's "eaves." The edge you are rolling

tightly becomes the handle.
The rat-tail should finish in a
nice taper, with the bulk of the
weight in this rolled handle.
Wet the tip, and look out.

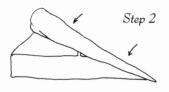

Step 2

Warning, this is no toy. It is as dangerous as a single-tail.
Well, almost. But it is one of the few toys you can wipe up
with when you are through playing.

Of course, there are substitutes for the leather and metal
accoutrements of your boudoir that travel easily and incon-
spicuously. I have already mentioned plastic tie wraps and
Saran Wrap. You can also use Saran Wrap to make a wonderfully camp fetish outfit, including a corset that really
works quite well. Nothing looks too suspicious about that
utilitarian and tacky binder, duct tape (unless, of course, it is
in a bag with a ski mask, rope, and a revolver). And it is
handy to have for other eventualities, too, like that slit in
your checked luggage from the baggage people trying to get at
your toys. Duct tape is not very forgiving to skin, though. It
is as much a depilatory as a bondage resource.

What if you are in your four-star hotel room and you discover there are no St. Andrew's crosses in the guest-services
brochure? No problem, simply borrow a bellman's cart. Slip
the bellhop a couple of extra bucks after he has delivered your
luggage and promise to bring it downstairs when you finish.
Of course, if you want to borrow his pillbox hat, it will be a
few dollars more. The bellman's cart makes a wonderful
rolling stage from which to tie or suspend subbie. It is especially useful if he is blocking your view of the TV—you can
just roll him out of the way into a corner.

"as we make our final approach"

Remember, a little resourcefulness is a good thing. Perception is key to looking at your surroundings as useful tools for your D/s pleasure. Whether or not you came prepacked and prepared to capture, restrain, and titillate your (possibly newfound) playmate, you can usually make do by keeping your eyes open to the possibilities that surround you and by using your imagination.

d/tails: packing—as good as it gets

Besides whiskers on kittens, these are a few of my favorite things. Be sure some of these items make it into your bag.

A LEATHERMAN, or one of those multitool pliers contraptions, can be invaluable, and a great addition to your Swiss Army knife (the one with the corkscrew). The needle-nose pliers will help get knots out, and if you have to take the Gordian approach, there is always the knife blade. Don't be alarmed, the corkscrew is just for opening wine.

A SMALL FLASHLIGHT helps you find handcuff keys in those dark dungeons and hotel rooms.

A PLASTIC SQUEEZE BOTTLE filled with a 10 percent solution of chlorine bleach, for wiping down equipment after use. Put the plastic bottle inside of a Ziploc bag, and then put that into another Ziploc to prevent a nasty accident. You can easily look like a Holstein if you get a big white splotch on your black leather.

A FLASK OF VODKA. A decent sterilizing agent in a pinch, and also useful as a libation for those *après*-room-service hours. Better tasting by far than the chlorine solution mentioned above. After a session, I soak my ball gags in a glass of vodka (the Popov, not the Ketel One). The colored balls look like clown dentures.

ANOTHER PLASTIC SQUEEZE BOTTLE filled with a solution of one part glycerin and three parts water, to soothe skin after spanking and flogging. Put it in the Ziploc with the bleach solution. Also put in your Ziploc a bottle of tincture of arnica. When added to a washcloth with cool water it will inhibit bruising, although you should never use it on broken skin or internally.

SEVERAL PAIRS OF LATEX SURGICAL GLOVES. You can put them over plugs and vibrators for protection. They are more economical than condoms (which, by the way you should also pack). Latex gloves are great for naughty nurse/kinky doctor scenes. The gloves can also be filled with ice to use for ice packs; they can even be filled with water and frozen that way (a great way to chill punch at your dungeon parties). Oh yes, they work well as gloves, too.

CLOTHESPINS. Besides being delicious torture on soft body parts, they can also hang up your wet panties.

DUCT TAPE. Functional and kinky—form following

fetish. Put it in a Ziploc of its own so glue residue won't end up on your Chanel blouse. You can get small-diameter rolls so it doesn't take up so much space in your bag.

A SMALL FIRST-AID KIT, with Neosporin, Band-Aids, Q-Tips, and insurance cards, because one never knows.

NAIL CLIPPERS. A ragged nail can wreak havoc on expensive stockings and do even worse damage to latex, including condoms.

RIBBON AND SHOELACES. Get leather shoelaces in bulk from an outlet like Tandy. Inexpensive and very handy in tender places.

LUBRICATION. Put a spare tube in your makeup kit.

A TUBE OF SUPERGLUE. A domme friend of mine carried this in her fetish bag. I never once saw her use it, but it never failed to inspire terror in every male sub she ever had.

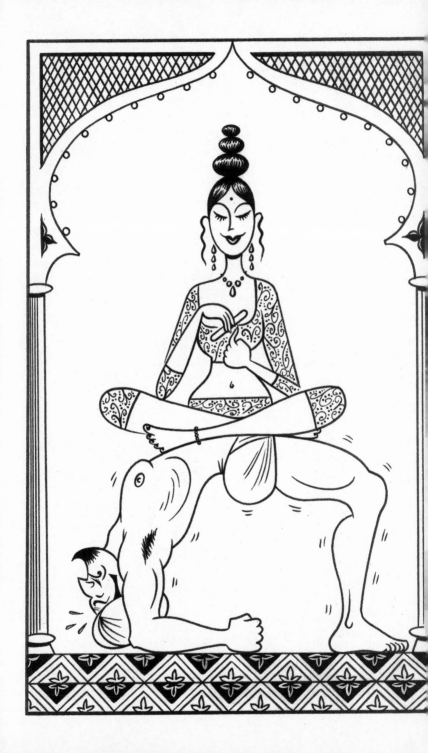

- 11 -

FIT TO BE TIED

workouts for tops and bottoms

Lovemaking, even in its most vanilla form, is an athletic endeavor. Imagine how high the cardiovascular bar is raised when you add a lockerful of whips and chains. Bondage itself is a workout. Like any other strenuous activity, a little exercise can enhance performance, and also the end result will be a buffer subbie and mistress.

Some of the best exercises are the stretching routines of yoga. Many of these positions, or *asanas,* are great guidelines for bondage poses. These are by no means all of the yoga exercises available, just the ones I think will enhance bondage, and symbiotically, will be enhanced by bondage. With or without rope, the following exercises will increase the strength and flexibility of your lover and quite possibly, your love.

kinkyoga

embryo and half tortoise balasana

Start in a prone position and inhale. As you exhale, bend your knees, curl your back, and pull your buttocks back toward your heels. Bring both arms to your sides and allow

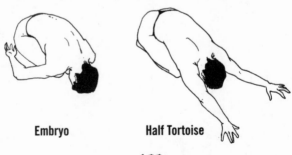

Embryo   **Half Tortoise**

your shoulders to droop in a totally passive, submissive position. This is the embryo. If you instead keep your arms extended on the floor, like "you are not worthy," then it is the half tortoise. These two are good starting positions and resting positions, and very good for the back, especially after a rigorous bow tie. It also affords the slave a good angle to admire your pedicure.

standing cobra and standing cat

Stand with your feet apart, inhale, and interlace your fingers behind your back, as if they were tied. With your knees slightly bent and your butt tucked under, slowly bring your hands up behind your back as high as they will go. Arch backward as you look up. Hold and breathe. This is the Standing Cobra. To reposition to the Standing Cat, release your hands

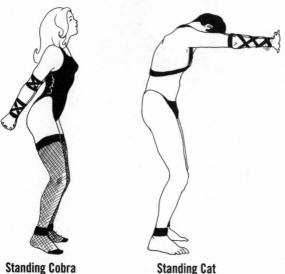

Standing Cobra   **Standing Cat**

and interlace the fingers in front of you, palms facing outward, with the elbows straight. Push harder as you exhale, trying to flatten your abdomen, with your head bent down in a submissive pose.

dog stretch: adho mukha svanasana

The perfect low stretch to show off your new dog collar is the dog stretch. From down on your hands and knees, inhale, curl your toes under, and begin to lift off your knees and raise your tailbone toward the ceiling. While pressing the heels down, stretch the straightened arms while bending the torso toward the floor, exhaling on the way. A great stretch for the back, even if it makes you feel like chasing a few cars.

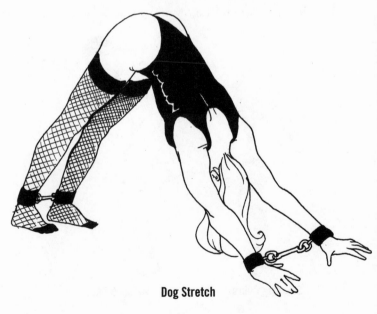

Dog Stretch

staff pose: dandasana

Although this doesn't look like much, this is a very dynamic seated position. Sit down with your feet straight out and your back ramrod straight. Put your arms a little behind your trunk and shoulder width apart, with fingers facing forward and palms flat on the floor. Push down hard on the palms while you thrust your chest out. Bury your chin on your chest and arch the toes back. Imagine your legs tied at the ankles and knees, and your arms tied at the elbows. This strengthens the back, tones the arms, stretches the hamstrings, and gets those elbows just a little closer. Another advantage is you can do this one and still watch a video.

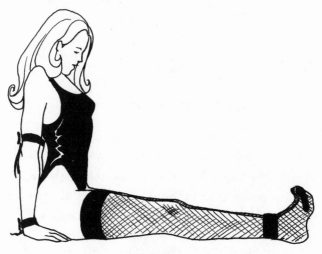

Staff Pose

yoga mudra

This begins in the lotus posture, the classic meditation pose with the legs crossed severely, each foot on the opposite thigh. Interlace your fingers behind the back, straighten your elbows, and lean forward, bringing your arms up in the air. With practice, your forehead will be on the floor and your arms pointing straight up.

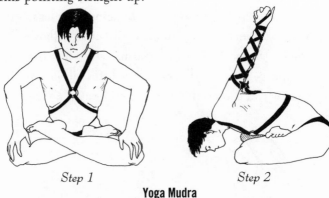

Step 1   *Step 2*

Yoga Mudra

locust pose: salabhasana

This is a hot pose for hands tied in front. Begin on the floor in a prone position, lying on your arms, which are straight with hands balled into fists, the wrists crossed and pressed together near the pelvis. Begin to lift your legs, which should be straight and pressed together, from your pelvis, while arching the back. Your weight is mainly on your forearms. With subbie's hands tied to a crotch rope, this is wonderfully confining.

Locust Pose

172

camel pose: ushtrasansa

Get on your knees (always a great place to start), lean back, and grab your right ankle with your right hand and your left ankle with your left hand. Keep the thighs straight and arch your back. Point your chin in the air. With your partner facing you in the same pose, it is possible to make love like this—tied or not.

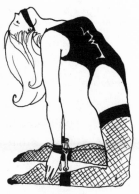

Camel Pose

the bow: dhanurasana

This is a great bondage posture and the namesake I use for what most everyone else calls the hog-tie. It is easier to do if you have first practiced with the camel pose. Lie on your stomach with your arms at your side. Reach back with the right hand and grab the right ankle, and follow suit on the left side. Raise your trunk and knees, gently but firmly pulling on each ankle, curving upward like, well, a bow. Although the sensation is intense, try to hold the pose for at least five seconds, and with practice, longer. Imagine being tied this way.

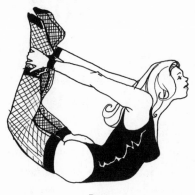

Bow

173

back stretch: pashchimatanasana

After doing an intense backward bend like the bow, it is good to alternate to a forward bending pose. The back-stretching pose works well for this, and is just the exercise to practice getting in a position where the hands can be tied to the feet while keeping the knees straight. Lie on your back with the arms outstretched above the head. Inhale deeply, and while holding the breath bend at the pelvis and sit up, keeping the head between the outstretched arms. Breathe out as you bend forward and continue to go down until the ankles can be grabbed. The head will end up on or near the knees. This is one that is actually easier if the subject is tied. Imagine the forearms tied to the lower legs and wrists tied to matching ankles. A rope can be put over the back and around the upper legs to tie the trunk to the legs.

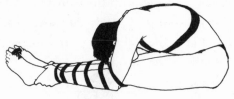

Back Stretch

forward bend: uttanasana or padahastasana

This pose, a human bobby pin of standing genuflection, is quite the workout for the hamstrings. Standing straight with your feet together, inhale. As you exhale, bend at the torso while keeping the knees straight. Your palms should eventually be flat on the floor on the outside of your feet, so

174

that your wrists could be tied to your ankles. Your head should be very close to your knees. Unless you have had special training, don't expect to do this one perfectly at first. For those of you into more advanced strap-on play, it is a great position for rear entry.

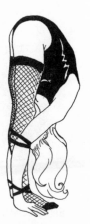

Forward Bend

headstand: sirshasana

You can tell by the word "sir" in the name of this asana that it is a master posture. This topsy-turvy stance is best practiced against a wall, or with leg manacles helping out over a bar. It will certainly help subbie get used to any advanced suspension techniques. Begin on your knees and interlace your fingers behind the head, separating your elbows by a forearm's width. Bend over as you exhale and place the bottom of your forearms, and the top of your head, on a pad on the floor. Your head and both elbows form an equilateral triangle. Inhale and straighten your legs and walk your buttocks up in the air. At some point your balance will equalize and the legs can be swung (or hoisted, if you are so inclined) above your head. Subbie's wrists can be loosely tied, but handcuffs on this one are dangerous. The blood rush to his head can be powerful, as can the up-close view of your Manolo Blahniks.

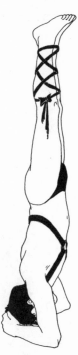

Headstand

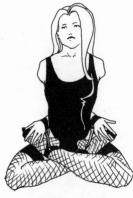

Bound Lotus Pose

bound lotus pose: baddhapapdmasana

If there is any doubt about the connection between kink and kundalini, then please check the translated name of this "badd" boy. Take a very vanilla lotus pose and cross the hands behind the back. Reach around and grab the left great toe in the left hand and the right great toe in the right. Being tied this way is absolute punishment. Twist and shout.

breathing for corsetry: pranayama

Part of the science of yoga is its ability to aid in the achievement of certain positions using the breath and breathing techniques. One place this can really come in

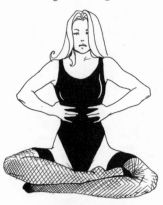

Breathing for Corsetry

handy is when you try to lace your subbie, or yourself, into one of the most delicious accessories in fetish wear, the corset. Different levels of pranayama deal with breathing from three different areas of the body: the abdomen, the lower rib cage, and the upper lung area near the collarbone. This exercise involves emptying your lungs completely and pulling in the abdomen as hard as you can, pulling in on the same areas a corset would push in. Hold for five seconds (or longer if you can). You can also use Saran Wrap as an aid to this exercise. Each time you exhale, wrap another tight layer of plastic around your abdomen. Seventeen inches is looking easier all the time, Scarlett.

whip-hand exercises

Swinging a flogger for even the shortest training session is surprisingly hard work. You can train for endurance and also rid yourself of that "I've got a bingo!" underarm flab by practicing with a five-pound weight. Stand comfortably (or, if in heels, uncomfortably) and, with the weight balanced in your whip hand and the opposite arm counterbalancing, slowly straighten your arm out in front parallel to the floor and at a right angle to your body, while you exhale, and slowly bend it back. Do three sets of fifteen repetitions, then switch arms and repeat. Now try the real thing and the whip or flogger will feel like a feather.

pony training

There exists an entire subculture of equestrian emulation called pony training, complete with such stable accessories as bridles, blinders, and harnesses. The high high-heeled kicks and prances that a prospective pony must do are an incredible aerobic workout that makes for healthy horsing around. And afterward, how nice to be brushed down with a curry comb. Giddy-up!

saran wrap undulation

This form of play doubles as a decent aerobic workout. Use the shrink roller to completely wrap your subbie. Have him comfortably in the middle of a large bed, or better yet a large pad or mattress on the floor. You may have to induce the wavelike motion with a few well placed crop taps to his buttocks, but the trick is to make him undulate like a worm. Advanced players can try to slither like an serpent. An apple gag completes the scene and Mistress Eve gets some long-overdue revenge. Bad snake.

just for feet

If you wish to move past starter stilettos, the proper exercises to increase the muscular strength in your feet and legs can be invaluable.

STRETCHING EXERCISES

1. For Achilles tendon and calf muscles: Stand facing a wall, an arm's length away. Rest your hands on the wall and lean forward, keeping your knees straight and heels flat on the floor. Use a small inclined plane for additional stretch.
2. A tried and true exercise skiers may have heard of: Stand on a platform about two inches high; phone books work well for this. Put the balls of your feet at the edge of the platform, as you would if you were doing a back dive from a diving board. Slowly drop your heels toward the ground until you feel a pull, then raise them back until they are

even with the platform. Increase the number of these you do as your calves and ankles get stronger.

STRENGTHENING EXERCISES

1. Sitting with your knees straight, bend your foot up and down slowly. Hold for two to five seconds.
2. Sitting with your knees bent, turn your foot in and out slowly.
3. Sit and slowly circle your feet.
4. Barefooted, sit on a towel on the floor, your knees bent enough so that you can grasp the towel with your toes. Curl your toes over the towel repeatedly, and pull it toward you, gathering it under your feet.
5. Stand with your feet parallel, six inches apart. First place your weight on the outer borders of your feet and then on the inner borders.
6. Stand with your feet parallel, four inches apart. Rise up on your toes and then swing your heels outward.
7. Stand with your feet parallel, three inches apart. Slowly rise on your toes and then rock into your heels.
8. Sit on a chair with your knees bent, lower legs crossed and feet resting on the outer borders. Curl your toes while you are seated in this position.
9. Walk on tiptoe, toes turned in, crossing your feet.
10. Sit on a chair with one ankle over the knee of the opposite leg. Bend your foot up and down slowly, applying resistance with your hands. Reverse legs and repeat.
11. While seated in the same position as step 10, turn your foot in and out, giving resistance with your hand. Reverse legs and repeat.

12. Lie down and put a strap under your forefoot, holding both ends of the strap with your hands. Pull up on the strap as hard as you can while your foot resists and pushes down, curling your toes down.

PAMPERING

1. Before a long stretch of wearing heels, rub your feet with lotion and put cotton socks on, sleeping this way for three nights in a row. It will help make your feet softer and more yielding to the leather.
2. Silicone pads inside your shoes at the balls of your feet can help make your feet feel much more comfortable.
3. Lamb's wool, which you can find at dance supply stores, can help alleviate some of the problems associated with cramped toes when you separate the toes and pad in between them.

cool down

These exercises can add enjoyment to your sex life, and especially rigorous S & M lovemaking, by getting you and your slave in better shape. If physical fitness is already a part of your normal routine, then just as in your sex life, a little S & M can put life into your workout, too—like a leather carrot at the end of your treadmill. Even without the ropes, a good bondage mind-set—thinking how the stretches help you get into positions that were impossible at first—will make the effort feel a bit more worthwhile. When you do break out the bonds, you will be much more confident and comfortable. The end results will be to tie for.

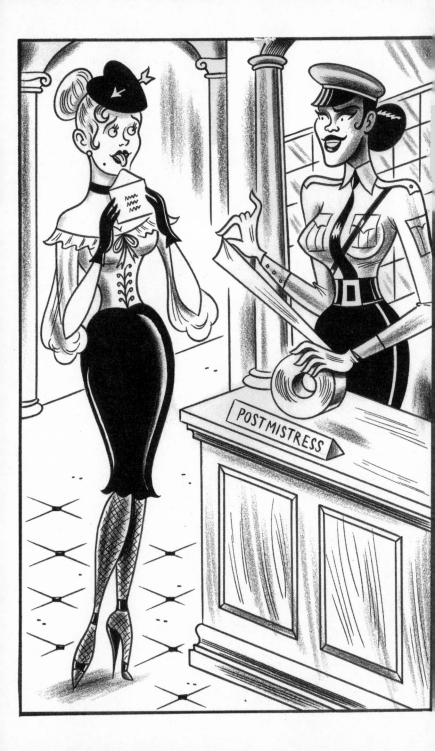

- 12 -

ANONYMOUSLY FREE TO BE YOU

looking for love
in all the write places

The awful daring of a moment's surrender, which an age of prudence can never retract. By this and only this we have existed.

—T. S. ELIOT

You have read this far, your interest is piqued, and maybe you've gone out and bought a few yards of rope or a pair of handcuffs. Now you must decide if, and how, you wish to begin to express and explore this aspect of your personality. Fortunately, you live in the nineties and have the opportunity to dip your toes in the springs of sexuality at your own pace and with minimal personal risk.

through the looking glass

If you decide to look to clubs or other venues to sate your desire to experience the world of dominance and submission, there are several ways to find a suitable partner with corresponding kinks. While talk TV could lead us to believe the country has a high-heel fetishist on every street corner and transvestites in an extraordinary number of Daughters of the American Revolution chapters, most social circles frown as much upon the open discussion of one's sexual preferences as they do idle speculation on Uncle Harold's genetic background. Personal ads in newspapers or regional magazines, communicating with online services (via bulletin board correspondence or real time conversation), nightclubs with fetish or S & M themes (like New York City's Hellfire), as well as local D/s organizations, are all viable options for finding your perfect play partner.

There has been much discussion about which of these avenues is the best for one to begin exploration. Some people will argue that there is no substitute for the experience of sitting and meeting others face-to-face. However, making the transition between realizing you have always enjoyed watching John Wayne tan the derriere of Maureen O'Hara more than most people to sitting in a room full of like-minded people is a big step. For this reason, meeting people through either the Internet or a newspaper ad is often a good transitional step.

do the write thing

Meeting people through personal ads in newspapers, magazines, or, increasingly, the Internet is a way of safely and anonymously expressing your desires and availability.

"It was in the April issue of *Washingtonian* that his ad first caught my eye," gushed Dale over lunch at the Palm. "Its headline was 'I Will Make You Accountable' and it read, 'CFO at a prestigious local company has a healthy appreciation for slide rules and their application on ladies who seek assistance in keeping a neat ledger.' I wrote to him and we corresponded for a week or two before we spoke on the phone, and we eventually met about two months after our initial exchange."

Dale's description of finding her dream dom through the personals section of a fine regional magazine is a wonderful testament to how two people can use the best of the resources the nineties have to offer to find a relationship more valuable than Park Avenue property. It should be noted that *time,* an invaluable ingredient in spicing up a succulent relationship, was used in order to create a critically important environment of personal and emotional safety.

the written word

Careful wording and good writing skills are the foundation of written communication. Writing frees you to express desires or feelings you might not ordinarily share, like my secret penchant for Beanie Babies. It also gives you the opportunity to edit and refine your thoughts before sharing them, thus eliminating the fear you might blurt out something foolish. The written word also allows the reader a chance to digest what he has read and formulate an informed opinion before responding.

Online correspondence affords participants many of the benefits of the traditional postal service without the need to moisten a stamp, and it also lessens the likelihood your letter will end up in some stranger's mailbox in Duluth. Most online services and Internet providers offer a chance for people to engage in real-time typewritten conversation. This form of communication allows you the benefits of virtually instantaneous feedback, but still gives you some time to measure your words before dispatching them.

Success in online communication requires the participants to have an ability to express themselves clearly through the written word. This is an excellent time to flaunt those good grades in expository writing at Swarthmore. Speed and accuracy in typing are also important for a fulfilling online conversation, the entire mood of which can be altered by the simple misplacement of an *o* or *i*.

After breaking the ice with your correspondent, you may want to exchange photographs. Stick to simple clothing and settings; the point is to show *you,* not the Delmarva beach house you stayed at last summer. It's fun to splurge and treat yourself and him to some glamour-shot photography, but remember there is a fine line between artistic embellishment and deliberate disingenuousness.

If your online D/s interactions turn to role-playing and other forms of creative writing, remember that attention to detail is extremely important, as is a good imagination. Dominants should be as descriptive as possible in setting the scene and issuing instructions. Creative inconsistencies such as ordering a submissive to get up and fix you a drink after you have just tied her to a rack will spoil the mood. However, having her hop on bound heels to the side bar is not only permissible, but recommended. Submissives should always respond politely, promptly, and in turn.

Becoming more and more popular is the use of small digital cameras. Connected to the monitor of your computer, these cameras allow you to see others via video transmissions that are very close to real time.

Pagers, which are increasingly inexpensive, lightweight, and versatile, can also be part of an electronic relationship. Numeric codes can be used to issue simple assignments or just to let the other person know you are thinking about her: for example, the number 7334 spells "hEEL" upside down. Vibrating pagers can also add a quick thrill to the tedium of any ordinary day, although special attention should be given to hiding the bulge they make when clipped to one's unmentionables.

why a nice girl like you should be in a place like this—bdsm clubs and organizations

Thus I reel from desire to fulfillment and in fulfillment languish for desire.
—GOETHE

Many major cities have D/s clubs that are usually open only on weekends. Attending one can be a good way for a neophyte to get a good sense of what the realities of sado-masochism are. Not only can you to compare your fantasies to the reality of different kinds of D/s play, but it can afford you the opportunity to meet other people who share your predilections. If you are looking for a partner with specific leanings, sometimes these places can be a good place to start.

It should also be noted that many large cities also have organizations whose members have a common interest in D/s. These organizations provide demonstrations, sponsor parties, and offer a wide range of other activities. Most of these groups advertise in alternative weekly newspapers or have information available on the Internet.

submissives, beware

Great care should be taken as you prepare to make the move from indirect to direct encounters. While most people make this move with no ill consequences, horror stories of people who lacked suitable judgment abound. Great care should be taken when setting up your initial meeting with a potential partner, just as you would be cautious about meeting any person for the first time.

Do not be shy about asking a dominant for references and information down to his golf handicap. Anyone worth his crop will understand your concerns and the reasons why you are doing this, and he certainly will not think any less of you. If he does have a problem with it, I would advise you to seek elsewhere or put your favorite Pinkerton to work in order to ensure that the condo in Cozumel is as legitimate as his season tickets to the Met. Of course, there are instances where a dominant will also be new and so will have no references. While learning together can be fun, there are inherent dangers in this, and a new dom must practice and study the application of the techniques he plans on using on his submissive. Remember, an overeagerness to get into stocks and bonds can be as bad as jumping the gun to get out of them.

Be sure the expectations that you have for a relationship match those of your prospective partner. Honesty is critical. A submissive who tells a dominant she only wants a bi-monthly spanking when what she really wants is a man to settle down and have children with, is creating major problems down the road. Or, if you are someone who requires a lot of attention, associating with a Mistress who has a large stable of studs is probably not for you.

Keep your hormones and enthusiasm in check on a first date. By doing so, you will earn the respect of your prospective partner and, more important, guarantee your safety. If you feel you may be overwhelmed by temptation, be sure to arrange a call to a friend to let him know where you are, who you are with, and another time that you will call. (This is a good rule of thumb for anyone going on a blind first date.)

I would also like to caution that female dominants, despite their titles and accoutrements, can sometimes be at risk. I advise that especially at a first-time play meeting, they take the time to go through the same safety precautions I advise submissives to go through.

People who are into bondage run a higher risk than others and should be extra careful. Never allow yourself to be gagged at a first-time play encounter. Never submit to any kind of locking devices. Never, under any circumstances whatsoever, should you allow yourself to be left alone.

do diligence

Just as today every niche of the social register has those with trust funds and those without, so it is too that all varieties of services will attract people who won't ever be able to tell a Montrachet from a Châteauneuf-du-Pape. At these times, you must have the fortitude to make yourself a dry Absolut martini with a twist and assure yourself that with diligence and the application of the standards you have worked all your life to cultivate, you will find the fulfillment you have been looking for.

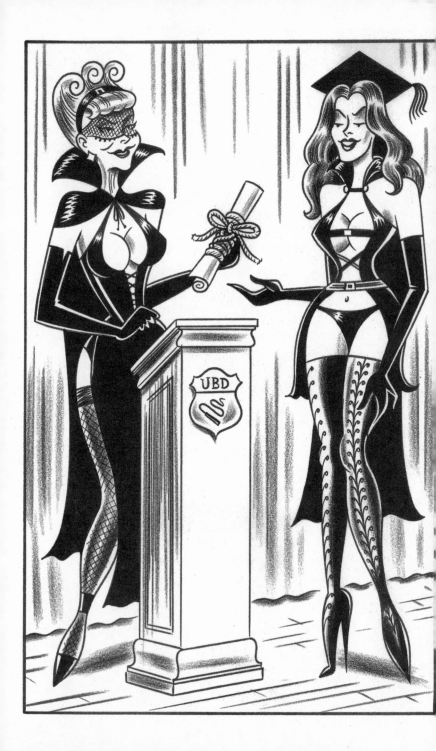

- 13 -

OFF THE
BEATEN PATH

advanced activities

If the thought of tying up and whipping your partner has become your idea of the usual Saturday night, now is the time to consider adding some unusual play activities and equipment to your command of kink.

Special care must be taken with these activities, which run the gamut from messy to dangerous. But this shouldn't deter you, as the precautions necessary to make it a night to remember (and not fifteen to twenty behind bars) are as practical as those for safely operating a motor vehicle.

wax

As easy as it is to cover your submissive with affections, it is equally easy to cover him with wax or liquid latex. While your love may have no bounds, it is best to confine your play with these materials to an area covered with a plastic tarp. This will allow you to protect the things you really care about, like the newly varnished floor or grandmother's antique quilt.

You will also want to take some measures to ensure the comfort of your bottom. Wax and liquid latex will both remove body hair faster than you can say Sinéad O'Connor, and most people are not enthusiastic about the prospect of having their hair ripped out by the roots, unless it is around the bikini-line area. Clearly, the only option is to begin your work on a smooth surface, so take out your razor and get to it.

If shaving is out of the question, you can try coating his skin with Lubriderm and then have him wear a body stocking or nylons, depending on where your artistic leanings take you, but this method is not 100 percent effective. Before coating him, make a little test area on an inconspicuous spot and see how much of a problem his body hair will be. Generally, the coarser and thicker the hair, the more likely it is to stick to wax or latex. If your partner is a woman, body-hair concerns are not as great as those for men, but if you don't know if her pubic area is shaved, make sure to ask ahead of time. The sound a submissive makes when wax-coated panties are being ripped off the Devil's Triangle is best described as bone-chilling—so again, be sure to ask.

While your natural inclination may be to buy the finest of beeswax candles to drip on your consort, he will receive your objective much more happily if you purchase inexpensive candles instead. Ironically, some of the best candles for waxing poetic are the kosher candles easily found around Passover and Hanukkah. The wax from these candles melts at a very low temperature, which means it is less likely to burn the skin. Very fine wax, like beeswax, burns very fast and very hot, as does dark wax, like black or navy blue. Scented candles will also burn at a higher temperature than unscented ones. Fetish shops often carry special candles designed for waxing. Unlike the kosher candles, which are tapers, these specialty candles are often pillar style, which have a wider melting area, and therefore more wax.

The sensation of warm wax flowing over your body can be very erotic if you keep a few things in mind. First, the greater the distance between the wax and your target, the cooler the wax will be. However, this distance will cause spattering and affect your accuracy, so be especially careful that wax intended for the chest does not end up on the neck or face.

Don't concentrate the wax all in one area. Begin by drizzling it over as much of your submissive as you intend to cover. As you add layers, you can begin to play with the intensity of the heat of the wax by decreasing the distance, or by using a darker colored candle, which, as you will remember, burns hotter. Have a bucket of ice nearby to soothe the parched lips of your subbie and to provide a sharp contrast to the heat of the wax (or use it to make it harden faster).

Keeping your sub from developing unsightly wax buildup is easy enough. You can scrape most of it off with your fingernails, and any remaining residue is easily washed off in the shower.

liquid latex

> **Warning:**
> 1. Never cover the entire body with liquid latex—if the skin cannot breathe, it can be fatal.
> 2. Find out if your sub is allergic before using latex—an allergic reaction can be toxic or fatal.

Liquid latex provides a similar sensory experience to wax, except that it is cool. It also has unique qualities and special considerations. Liquid latex is literally a special type of latex paint that can be used almost anywhere on the body, and it comes in a variety of colors. If enough layers are applied, you can create a piece of custom-made latex clothing that can even be reused, if carefully removed. Be aware that such an endeavor takes a great deal of time and a lot of latex. Each layer takes about fifteen or twenty minutes to dry, and you will need at least half a dozen layers, applied according to manufacturer's instructions, to make a serviceable covering. A hair dryer can be used to speed this process, but unless you have an assistant or two, this does not seem to be a huge time saver.

Along with being messy, liquid latex has an ammonialike odor that is pretty nasty and that some people have an adverse reaction to. Combat this by creating your masterpiece in a well-ventilated area. These chemicals can also be harsh to sensitive skin, so be sure to try the latex on a small patch first. Also remember that liquid latex has many of the same chemical properties as latex in its solid form, so before beginning, ensure you partner does not have a latex allergy. And never cover the entire body; skin needs to be able to breathe.

Liquid latex is water soluble, so subbie will come clean with a little soap and water, and it won't harm your sewer pipes.

electrical play

Playing with electricity isn't for the faint of heart—literally. It is an absolute no-no if your subbie has a history of heart problems. Electrical devices should never be used above the waist, nor should they be used on any piercings. And of course, you never want to use the Violet Wand on your submissive when he is taking a bath, as he could be fatally electrocuted.

You should never buy any of these devices until you feel you are well versed in being able to read your bottom's responses to stimulation. You are playing with electricity, and while a slight twist of a knob will mean nothing to you, it can make all the difference between subbie heaven and subbie hell.

violet wands

One story is that the Violet Wand was invented in the fifties as a nerve stimulator to combat arthritis and related ailments. Another is that it was invented in the early 1900s as a quack cure for cancer and glaucoma (one of the attachments, which looks like a mushroom, was designed to fit over a closed eye). Later, the wand was used by certified cosmetologists to remove static from hair. The bottom line is, they've been around for a long time and really don't do any of these things, but they are a great tool if you are interested in playing with static electricity.

I think the most attractive thing about the Violet Wand is how it looks. When activated, the glass tubes become a luminescent purple and emit purple sparks. The purple glow comes from electricity passing through the ionized gas inside the glass and mirroring the gas's color—in this case, purple. Once static electricity passes through the glass tube, it passes into the atmosphere, making sparks and creating ozone, which serves a double purpose as an air purifier.

Dozens of attachments are available for your wand, but most sets come equipped with a maximum of six. Among the most notable are the aforementioned mushroom-shaped "eye attachment" and a long tube called "the concentrator" that is the most intense of commonly available options. My favorite is something called "Lightning Hands"—by holding it you become an electrical conductor. Do you have a shocking imagination?

The wand has a knob at the bottom of its base that allows you to control the intensity of the static electricity. If the wand is placed directly on the skin and contact is not broken, it pro-

duces a tingly, vibrating sensation, the extent of which is deter-
mined by the intensity selected. However, if you hold the Wand
about a quarter of an inch away from the skin, a focused
stream of static electricity is created, which results in consider-
ably more intense sensation. This stream will cease as soon as
contact with the skin is made again, or if the distance from the
wand to the skin is increased to more than a half an inch.

The problem with Violet Wands is twofold. The device is
very expensive (a deluxe unit with six attachments goes for
about $400) and it's one of those love it or hate it kinds of
things. Unless you are certain this is something you simply
must own, you may want to borrow one first and take it for a
test run before you spend that much money on something that
might be relegated to scaring the cats on a slow night at home.

TENS unit

TENS stands for *Transcutaneous Electrical Nerve Stimulator*.
A TENS unit is a small, battery-operated device that trans-
mits small electrical impulses through the skin to the under-
lying peripheral nerves.

While TENS units are common items found at BDSM
stores, I do **not** recommend them as part of your D/s toy
chest. However, if you are seized by an impulse of the non-
electrical kind and this item ends up in your shopping bag,
remember to never, ever, ever use it above the waist, as it can
cause fatal defibrillation of the heart muscle.

EPILOGUE

There is nothing more satisfying to this domme's ears than that little moan of satisfaction, the little silenced sigh, that escapes from my slave when my pleasure is his. I would like to think as you complete this introduction to D/sneyland that you are unleashing a similar sigh of satisfaction.

Or perhaps I hear a *click* instead, as some hidden aspect of your personality switches on, giving you new ideas for surprising your partner this Saturday night.

If nothing else, you are better informed, and even if you choose not to use any of these tips, maybe they will be fantasy fodder for the next time you hear the box springs creaking with the sound of business as usual.

You have my permission to let a little wicked smile play over your lips as you think about what you could be doing.

You do not have permission, however, to be offended by my predilection. BDSM is a tool for creating intimacy in your relationship, not an amoral vice of the damned. It is a dash of cayenne in the broth—a bit of cinnamon in the potpourri. The unique yin-yang of sexuality and power exchange in D/s touches on two of our most ingrained instincts—no wonder so many of us find the subject exciting and intriguing.

You also do not have permission to be careless or foolish. Another part of S&M's appeal is the danger, but *looking* dangerous is enough. If you follow my tips with care and safety in mind, you can avoid D/saster. As I have emphasized in these proceeding chapters, all it takes to have the world of BDSM at your command is a sincere interest in creating a sexual environment that is as safe and as thrilling as your favorite carnival ride.

Epilogue

Take what you have learned here and use it to your advantage, whether you simply use the appeal of the heel, or a good square knot. Have fun with it. Be as domme as you want to be, and the next sound you may hear could be, "Thank you, Mistress, may I have another?"

APPENDIX

roaming on the web

books

http://www.apocalypse.org/circlet/home.html
http://www.qualitysm.com
http://www.amazon.com
http://www.thepoint.net/~pastpat/corset patterns

crafts

http://www.frugaldomme.com
http://www.cuffs.com

general information

http://gloria-brame.com/subbook.html
http://alternate.com/
http://www.cis.ohio-state.edu/hypertext/faq/usenet/FAQ-
    List.html
http://www.columbia.edu/cu/cv/others/asbwel1.html
http://www.mcsp.com/tes/welcome.html
http://www.yahoo.com/Society_and_Culture/
http://www.cyberzaar.com/dscuss
http://www.MJsLeathernet.com

shopping

http://www.zoom.com/divanet/erotica2
http://www.centurians.com
http://www.northbound.com

Appendix

corsets

http://www.lechatexotique.com
http://www.romantasy.com
http://www.starkers.com
http://www.divaweb.com

shoe shopping and information

http://www.iconet.com.br/~elizalde/shoes/

whips

http://www.catalog.com/utopian/catalog/ index.html

spanking information

http://www.shadowlane.com

metal clothing and accessories

http://www.sblades.com

handcuffs

http://www.blacksteel.com

You have permission to contact Mistress Payne at
http://www.MistressPayne.com